PREVENTING DIABETES

Learn how you can prevent becoming diabetic or if you are already diabetic, learn the best way to control or even possibly reverse your diabetes.

D1167134

Ray D. Strand, M.D.

Every effort has been made to make this book as accurate as possible. The purpose of this book is to educate. It is the review of scientific evidence, which is presented for information purposes. No individual should use the information in this book for self-diagnosis treatment, or justification in accepting or declining any medical therapy for any health problems or diseases. Any application of the advice herein is at the reader's own discretion and risk. therefore, any individual with a specific health problem or who is taking medications must first seek advice from their personal physician or health care provider before starting a nutritional program. The author and Health Concepts Publishing shall have neither liability nor responsibility to any person or entity with respect to loss, damage, or injury caused or alleged to be caused directly or indirectly by the information contained in this book. We assume no responsibility for errors, inaccuracies, omissions, or any inconsistency herein. Any slights of people, places, or organizations are unintentional.

Printed in the United States of America

First printing 2006

ISDN 0-9664075-0-4

Creative: www.tmdesigns-slc.com

ATTENTION MEDICAL FACILITIES, CORPORATIONS, UNIVERSITIES, COLLEGES, AND PROFESSIONAL ORGANIZATIONS: Quantity discounts are available on bulk purchases of this book for educational purposes. Special books or book excerpts can also be created to fit specific needs. For information, please contact Real Life Press, P.O. Box 9226, Rapid City, SD 57709.

PART 1

PREVENTING OR REVERSING DIABETES

The Center for Disease Control (CDC) projected a couple of years ago that any child born after the year 2000 would have over a 30% chance of developing diabetes sometime during his or her lifetime. If the child happened to be Black, Hispanic, or Native American, the chance of developing diabetes would jump to nearly 50%. This would mean that every second or third person in this present, new generation would end up developing diabetes. Can you imagine or even fathom how this would affect the health, not only of these individuals, but our nation? When you consider that diabetes is not only the leading cause of adult blindness, amputations, kidney failure, and neuropathy, but also the major cause of premature death, you begin to see why this projection by the CDC is so very important. Is the die cast? Is there any hope? Are we simply going to be the victims of our genetics and the All-American and Western diet? Can diabetes be prevented or even reversed? Well, this is what this booklet is all about.

You have just now entered my exam room, and I am about to give you a personal consult to show you how you can prevent becoming diabetic over 90% of the time, even if you are genetically susceptible or already have early signs of diabetes. If you are already diabetic, I am also going to lay out the strategies that will allow you to tightly control your diabetes with minimal dependence on medication and, in some cases, even be able to eliminate medication altogether. Many of my type 2 diabetic patients have also been able to totally reverse their diabetes by applying these healthy lifestyles to their lives.

DIABETES MELLITUS

Type 1 Diabetes Mellitus or Juvenile Diabetes

I need to define the different types of diabetes mellitus so there is no confusion as to which type I am referring. Type I diabetes mellitus was initially referred to as juvenile diabetes. Most researchers believe that this type of diabetes is the result of an autoimmune response to a viral infection. Type 1 diabetes occurs almost exclusively in children. Anytime you have an autoimmune response, the immune system basically begins attacking an organ or system of the body. In this case, the immune system begins attacking and destroying the beta cells of the pancreas where insulin is produced. After it destroys all of the beta cells, your body is not able to make insulin and your blood sugars begin to rise to very high levels. Unless you begin to receive insulin in some fashion right away, you cannot survive. Your body will require insulin injections the rest of your life. Now there are many different types of insulin and different ways to get it into the body; however, you will need to be taking some type of insulin to survive. Only 2 to 3% of all the diabetics in the world have type 1 diabetes mellitus.

You are not able to reverse this type of diabetes, unless of course, you have a pancreatic transplant. That is not as unusual as it seems. Some of the most successful transplants being done today are pancreatic transplants. I personally feel that over the next decade this procedure will become commonplace. Applying the principles that I share in this booklet will help you protect your arteries and decrease your risk of secondary complications due to your diabetes. This is critical when you consider that there is a good possibility of having a pancreatic transplant in your future. However, even if you do not have that opportunity, applying these principles to your life will allow you the absolute best chance of protecting your health and living into your old age.

Insulin Dependent Type 2 Diabetes Mellitus

Approximately 10% of the diabetics today fall into the category of insulin dependent, type 2 diabetes. This disease usually comes on during your adult years; however, the difference is the fact that your body just quits making insulin. No one really knows why, although there are several theories being tossed around. The key point is the fact that if you have insulin dependent diabetes, you will need insulin in some form to survive. You usually do not fit into the typical category of those individuals who develop type 2 or adult-onset diabetes. Most of these patients are thin, previously healthy individuals who much like the type I diabetics begin to complain about increasing thirst, frequent urination, unusual weight loss, and increasing fatigue. Physicians are usually surprised to see a significantly elevated blood sugar on the chemistry profile. Like the type I diabetics, the chances of complications due to their disease is significantly increased.

Again, if these individuals begin applying the principles shared in this booklet, they will present themselves with the best opportunity to avoid the secondary complications of their disease and protect their health. Since you produce very little or no insulin, you will not be able to actually reverse your diabetes. Your goal is to have excellent control of your diabetes so that you significantly reduce the complications due to your disease.

Type2 Diabetes Mellitus or Adult-Onset Diabetes

Over 90% of the individuals developing diabetes today develop type 2 diabetes or what was previously referred to as adult-onset diabetes mellitus. This type of diabetes normally takes decades to develop and is the most preventable form of diabetes. Over time these individuals become less and less sensitive to their own insulin. The body compensates for this situation by actually making more and more insulin to compensate for this insensitivity. As the blood insulin levels rise, the body is able to still control blood sugar levels. However, as you will learn a little later in this booklet, there are several metabolic changes that occur as soon as these blood insulin levels begin to rise even though your blood sugars still remain normal and you do not show any signs of diabetes. The moment you develop insulin resistance, your arteries begin to age much faster than they should.

As long as you are able to keep producing these abnormally high levels of insulin (hyperinsulinemia), your blood sugars will remain normal. However, over the years, in the overwhelming majority of cases, your body simply can't keep making all of this insulin. In the majority of individuals with this problem the insulin levels finally begin to drop. As these insulin levels begin to drop, your blood sugars will then begin to rise and you become diabetic.

You will learn that you don't just wake up one day and develop type 2 diabetes mellitus. There are all kinds of early warning signs that you are becoming insulin resistant and at high risk of developing diabetes in the very near future. In fact, in my practice I have learned to look for these signs that allow me to accurately predict who will most likely become diabetic 10 to 15 years before they actually become diabetic. It is during this time that my patients have the best chance of reversing their underlying insulin resistance, slowing down the aging process, and preventing the development of type 2 diabetes mellitus. These are the individuals who will benefit the most from the principles shared in this booklet because they can actually prevent becoming diabetic. Is it worth the effort? I will let you decide. However, I have found that the majority of patients who realize that they are in the early stages of developing diabetes are very willing to make the simple lifestyle changes necessary to improve insulin sensitivity. My job is to present the medical evidence that supports this claim and the 12 years of clinical experience in accomplishing this goal in my private family practice.

The Metabolic Syndrome

The metabolic syndrome, or what has also been referred to as the insulin resistance syndrome or syndrome X, is a constellation of problems that develops because of underlying insulin resistance. Please refer to Table 1 to see a list of problems that may develop when you become less and less sensitive to your own insulin.

From a clinician's point of view, I have personally observed hundreds of patients over the years that have slowly developed the many problems associated with the silent threat of the metabolic syndrome. Even though I only became aware of insulin insensitivity and its effects to the health of my patients approximately twelve years ago, I have since reviewed past physical exams and blood work for patients who have been in my care over the past three decades. I've conducted annual physicals for

TABLE 1
Metabolic Syndrome—A Constellation of Serious Problems

• Central Obesity	• Increased Fibrinogen Levels
• High Blood Pressure	• Increased Risk of Cardiovascular Disease
• Elevated Triglyceride Level	• Polycystic Ovarian Disease
• Increased Risk of Diabetes	• Increased VLDL Cholesterol Level
• Low HDL "good" Cholesterol Level	

the police, sheriff, fire departments, and the majority of my patients. Therefore, I have archives of documented results (longitudinal studies) of the gradual changes in individuals' health status over a long period of time in patients who actually developed insulin resistance and diabetes.

What I have discovered is that full-blown metabolic syndrome does not just develop all of a sudden. It comes as the result of years and years of daily choices and poor lifestyles. A sedentary lifestyle along with the All-American diet has caused a tremendous number of my patients to develop the metabolic syndrome and eventually type 2 diabetes. The number of people who are starting down this slippery slope of accelerated aging is mind-boggling. The Journal of the American Medical Association had a review article that stated that nearly 25% of the adult population already has the metabolic syndrome and many of our children are also developing this silent disease. What I have observed in my private clinical practice is the fact that another 25% of the population is on their way to developing insulin resistance. This means that about 50% of the adult population and nearly 1/3 of our children already have evidence of early insulin resistance or the full-blown metabolic syndrome. In fact, I am impressed when I find a patient who is not beginning to show signs of insulin resistance. The numbers are becoming fewer each year. Here is the astonishing part: **unlike a genetic disorder, this phantom syndrome can be fully prevented.** The earlier you reverse insulin resistance with the healthy lifestyles shared in this booklet, the greater your chance is of reversing any insulin resistance, preventing diabetes altogether, and protecting your health. Remarkably, this damaging process can be reversed at almost any stage along the way—even after becoming diabetic!

STAGES OF INSULIN RESISTANCE

It is critical for you to know exactly where you stand in the progression of this disease. Is this the reason you can't lose weight? Is this reason that you are developing high blood pressure or elevated cholesterol, or heart disease, or diabetes? This may be a health problem you need to address in your own life before it's too late? What will you do with the dangerous phantom lurking in the unseen corners of your life? We need to take a closer look at how this deadly syndrome develops. To do so, I have divided the development of the metabolic syndrome into four stages: abusing insulin, early insulin resistance, metabolic syndrome, and diabetes mellitus.

Stage I—ABUSING OUR INSULIN

We've been led to believe we are eating "healthy enough" when we try to watch the amount of fat we are consuming in our diet. The medical community has given its nod of approval to our bagel, cold cereal, instant oatmeal, toast, and sweetened orange juice, as a fine way to start our day. Along with white bread, white flour, potatoes, cereals, and rice these foods are known to spike your blood sugar very rapidly and as you will learn later in this booklet are referred to as high-glycemic carbohydrates. In fact, over 80 to 90% of the carbohydrates consumed by adults and children today are high-glycemic. This rapidly rising blood sugar significantly stimulates the release of insulin, your "storage" hormone. Insulin's job is to control blood sugar, which it does by driving the blood sugar into the cell to be utilized as energy or stored as fat or glycogen. What most people do not realize is the fact that this over stimulation of insulin results in the blood sugar

9

dropping almost as fast as it went up. It usually drops into the low blood sugar range or hypoglycemic range. This in turn stimulates the release of our stress hormones like adrenaline and cortisol. Yes, our blood sugar will slowly return to normal; however, we are left with an "uncontrollable hunger" that I refer to as a carbohydrate addiction. We have no choice. We will crave another meal or snack and it usually contains more high-glycemic carbohydrates so that this vicious cycle starts all over again.

With the continual spiking of blood sugar, we are literally abusing our insulin because we are over-stimulating its release several times each and every day. One of the most serious effects of abusing one's insulin is the damage that starts to take place in the arteries. The rapid rise in blood sugar following a high-glycemic meal or a can of soda, sports drink, or even sweetened fruit juice actually causes significant inflammation to the fine lining of our arteries (called the endothelium). This is the start of what is now believed to be the initial defect leading to insulin resistance.

Elevated sugar in the blood stream following an unhealthy meal is one of the major causes of inflammation to this fine lining of our arteries. This inflammation primarily affects the smallest arteries called capillaries in the muscle. This rapidly rising blood sugar is the cause of this inflammation and I now refer to this phenomenon as glycemic stress.

Glycemic Stress

I would like to introduce a new concept, which I refer to as "glycemic stress." This condition is primarily due to the increased number of free radicals created by these rapidly rising and elevated blood sugars. Most health care professionals are not aware that even a short-term, rapid rise in blood sugar causes stress to the fine lining of the arteries. This is particularly true in the capillaries or smallest arteries of the muscle. This glycemic stress occurs shortly following a high-glycemic meal when the blood sugars are rising rapidly. The initial insult to the artery is due to the increased production of these charged oxygen molecules, which are called free radicals. The oxidative stress that is created damages the fine lining of the capillaries. This repeated insult to the capillaries of the muscle is the beginning of insulin resistance.

Basically, when the lining of the artery becomes inflamed or dysfunctional, it has a tendency to constrict and thicken. This thickened arterial wall actually creates a physical barrier that makes it more difficult for insulin to leave the blood stream and pass into the fluid around the cell where it is able to attach to the insulin receptor sites on the surface of the cell—allowing sugar to be transported into the cell.

You must begin to realize what is happening to your arteries each and every time you indulge yourself with a meal loaded with processed and high-glycemic carbohydrates. Over the years of abusing your insulin, your arteries will become more and more thickened. Eventually you will "tip over" into this abnormal metabolic state we now refer to as the metabolic syndrome.

Stage 2—EARLY INSULIN RESISTANCE

Many theories abound as to why insulin resistance develops in certain individuals and not in others. Regardless of their differences, however, more and more studies are showing that endothelial dysfunction primarily in the capillaries of the muscle is an early and prominent event in the process.

Published research by Jonathan Pickney, et al. titled, "Endothelial Dysfunction: Cause of the Insulin Resistance," *Diabetes,* 1997, supports this theory. Pickney states that the endothelial dysfunction that causes insulin resistance primarily involves the smallest vessels that make up the capillary bed. This endothelial dysfunction created by high blood sugar and the high surges of insulin which follow (known as hyperglycemia and hyperinsulinemia), causes vasoconstriction (narrowing of the arteries), in the capillary bed. It has been demonstrated that a constricted and inflamed endothelium is actually a physical barrier to the transport of insulin to the insulin receptor sites of the muscle, adipose, and liver cells. The body responds to this situation by actually stimulating the beta cells of the pancreas to produce more and more insulin. In other words, the body tries to compensate for this insulin resistance by producing more and more insulin and basically hammering the insulin across this thickened arterial wall.

In this situation, insulin levels become *elevated* (hyperinsulinemia). *A person in this stage has now crossed the line from merely abusing his or her insulin to actually developing early signs of true insulin resistance.* As the blood insulin levels begin to rise, there are many metabolic changes that occur within the body that is now referred to as the metabolic syndrome. One's blood pressure begins to rise, the triglyceride levels and very bad LDL cholesterol increase, the good or HDL cholesterol begins to decrease, the individual starts gaining weight around their middle, and they are now are at high risk of developing heart disease and diabetes. This constellation of problems is what makes up the metabolic syndrome. **Once hyperinsulinemia develops, a chain of events is triggered that cannot be stopped without significant lifestyle changes.**

Some Important Definitions

HDL—the "good" cholesterol (should be above 40 in men and above 50 in women)—actually cleans up our arteries by transporting excess LDL cholesterol back to the liver.

Triglyceride—the other fat in your blood stream (usually should be less than 100)—is now becoming a major player in the development of coronary artery disease.

Triglyceride/HDL Ratio—the ratio that gives an indirect measurement of blood insulin levels—should be less than 2. The higher this ratio is the higher your blood insulin.

LDL—the "bad" cholesterol—causes significant inflammation to the arteries when it becomes oxidized by excessive free radicals.

VLDL—the very small, dense LDL cholesterol, which is much worse than its larger cousin the LDL cholesterol.

Lipotoxicity—the damage caused to the beta cell of the pancreas due to the high levels of fat in the blood stream.

Glucotoxicity—the damage caused to the beta cell of the pancreas due to high levels of blood sugar

As a physician, one of the first things I note regarding patients who are entering stage 2 insulin resistance, is a decrease in HDL or good cholesterol level (for women a score of below 50 (1.29 mmol/L), and for men below 40 (1.04 mmol/L), which is also associated with increasing triglyceride levels. This pattern is fairly typical for those just entering stage 2 insulin resistance and is evidence that the patient is developing insulin resistance. I calculate a simple ratio by dividing the patient's triglyceride level by their HDL cholesterol level. When the Triglyceride/HDL cholesterol level is greater than 2, I believe that my patients are starting to develop early insulin resistance. Since triglyceride levels begin to rise and the HDL cholesterol levels decrease as the blood insulin levels rise, this ratio is actually an indirect indication of the severity of their insulin resistance and of their blood insulin levels. The higher this ratio becomes the higher the patient's blood insulin levels. Therefore, in my office, I do not routinely do blood insulin levels because they tend to be fairly expensive and are not well standardized. Instead, I use the blood lipid profile, which is a common and an inexpensive test to order.

It is also during this stage that central obesity begins to develop, which is evidenced by an expanding waistline. I am now routinely measuring my patients' waistlines and documenting any increase. These observations along with the blood work allow me to determine which of my patients are just beginning to develop insulin resistance. Their arteries are already beginning to age much faster than they should and they are at a much higher risk of developing diabetes some 10 to 15 years down the road. Thus, offering these individuals the full opportunity to intervene and reverse this process before permanent and non-reversible damage has occurred to one's arteries is "True" preventive medicine. At this point, the patient is usually able to easily reverse his or her insulin resistance with the permanent healthy lifestyles I present in this booklet. They usually never go on to develop all the health consequences of the metabolic syndrome.

I have described some of the significant details of what is happening inside your body on a cellular and hormonal level. However, while this is taking place you may not "feel" any changes. You will most likely feel fine with few physical complaints other than feeling groggy or craving carbs. Patients may also begin to note increased nighttime eating and slowly increasing weight gain. This is why the phantom-like progression of insulin resistance is so dangerous.

The fact remains that most physicians do not even attempt to look for these early signs of insulin resistance and if they were to recognize them, most would not know what should be done to change its course. Why? I personally feel it is because we don't have a drug approved by the FDA for the early treatment of insulin resistance. Yet physicians are certainly ready and willing to treat the consequences that results from insulin resistance.

When I graduated from medical school and received my M. D. degree, I fully believed that I had become a "health care expert." After my intensive research of the medical literature during these past 10 to 12 years, I have begun to realize that I was actually a "disease care expert." I had been trained to recognize and treat disease. I wasn't trained to prevent anything. It is not surprising that physicians are trained to wait and treat the diseases that result from insulin resistance with their drugs. As you will learn, this is generally too late to prevent the diabetes and cardiovascular disease that is usually the result of this silent killer.

Stage 3—FULL-BLOWN METABOLIC SYNDROME

Over time, patients who have developed early insulin resistance become increasingly more resistant to their insulin, which causes insulin levels to continue rising higher and higher. These elevated insulin levels leads to dramatic metabolic consequences such as: high blood pressure, dyslipidemia, increased fibrinogen (blood clotting), cardiovascular disease, and diabetes.

Hypertension (high blood pressure)

One of the first signs of the full-blown metabolic syndrome, which is identified and treated by physicians, is the onset of high blood pressure. Insulin resistance, along with its resulting hyperinsulinemia, is known to increase the absorption of sodium from the kidneys, which causes a significant increase in fluid retention. This in turn increases one's blood pressure. High levels of insulin have also been shown to increase stimulation of our sympathetic nervous system, which causes additional constriction of the arteries and raises blood pressure. Insulin is also a potent growth factor and hyperinsulinemia abnormally stimulates the growth of the smooth muscles of the arteries. This also tends to cause one's blood pressure to rise.

Dyslipidemia

We have already discussed how the early signs of insulin resistance include the lowering of the HDL (good cholesterol) and the raising of triglycerides (fat particles). Continued high levels of insulin also stimulates the production the liver's production of VLDL (very-low-density lipoprotein) while at the same time causing a significant increase in the rate of breakdown of good cholesterol. This leads to the pattern so commonly seen in the metabolic syndrome of low HDL cholesterol, elevated triglyceride levels, and increasing levels of VLDL cholesterol—otherwise known as dyslipidemia. These tiny, dense LDL particles (VLDL) are very dangerous and cause further inflammation to the artery because they oxidize so easily.

Increased Fibrinogen Levels

Several proteins involved in the clotting process are affected by hyperinsulinemia. Fibrinogen, plasma plasminogen activator inhibitor 1, and several other clotting factors are elevated in those patients in stage 3 of the metabolic syndrome. This simply means that one tends to clot much more easily than they should. With all the problems that are now developing the risk for heart disease and stroke increases dramatically. In fact, Dr. Gerald Reavens, the leading authority in the metabolic syndrome, has stated that an individual who has the full-blown metabolic syndrome has over a 20-fold increased risk of a heart attack or stroke.

Cardiovascular Disease

Dyslipidemia, high blood pressure, hyperinsulinemia, elevated blood sugar levels, elevated fibrinogen, obesity, and the eventual diabetes that may develop are all independent risk factors for heart disease and stroke. A heart attack may be the first time you realize that you have a problem with insulin resistance. However, the unfortunate truth is that the first sign of heart disease over one third of the time is sudden death. **Premature death due to a heart attack or stroke is a major presentation of the metabolic syndrome.** The result of all these silent changes at the cellular level cuts off years from one's life.

The minute you begin to develop insulin resistance your arteries begin aging much faster than they should. It may take 10 to 15 years to actually develop diabetes; however, your arteries are being damaged much faster than normal as soon as you "tip over" into insulin resistance. This is why the day a physician actually diagnoses a patient as having diabetes, 60% of them already have major cardiovascular disease. It is a well-established fact that nearly 80% of our diabetic patients will die from a cardiovascular event like a heart attack or stroke. This was true in 1970 and it is true today. The medical community has not changed this terrible statistic in spite of all their new treatments and drugs that have been developed for the diabetic patient. The only way this statistic is going to change is by diagnosing insulin resistance in our patients earlier and guiding them into these new, healthier lifestyles that are known to improve insulin resistance.

Stage 4—DIABETES MELLITUS

The final outcome of the majority of patients with the metabolic syndrome is the development of type 2 diabetes mellitus, and in America this stage is being reached in epidemic proportions. **Type 2 diabetes mellitus has increased over 500% during the past generation with over 90% of these cases being due to insulin resistance.**

As long as the beta-cells of the pancreas are able to compensate for the ongoing state of insulin resistance by releasing excessive amounts of insulin, blood sugars will remain relatively normal. Over time, however, the beta cells of the pancreas simply wear out. As a result, blood sugars will now begin to rise and type 2 diabetes mellitus develops.

Individuals who suffer from the metabolic syndrome find themselves in a downward spiral that worsens over time. Two separate events must occur for those who develop type 2 diabetes mellitus (with the possible third factor of genetic predisposition). First, one obviously must have insulin resistance and second, one will have developed pancreatic beta cell exhaustion. Researchers now feel there is a combination of insults, which eventually lead to beta cell exhaustion and the decrease in insulin production. The chronic state of insulin resistance has required the beta cell to put out abnormally high amounts of insulin over time. As one's insensitivity to insulin worsens, the elevated levels of free fatty acids (lipotoxicity) along with slowly rising blood sugar levels (glucose toxicity) damage the beta cells and contribute to beta cell exhaustion.

Some people are genetically less susceptible to this damage to the beta cells. In fact, there are people who are able to continue producing high levels of insulin throughout their lifetime without ever becoming diabetic. As long as the body is able to compensate for one's insulin resistance by producing increased amounts of insulin, diabetes will not develop. **However, even though one does not develop diabetes, the accelerated aging of the arteries is still occurring due to the other metabolic changes associated with insulin resistance.**

SYMPTOMS AND SIGNS OF DEVELOPING INSULIN RESISTANCE

Stage 1—Insulin Abuse
- Fatigue and possibly shaky weakness following a meal
- Carbohydrate Cravings or an uncontrollable hunger (emotional eating)
- Pattern of nighttime eating
- Slowly increasing weight gain (expanding waist size)
- Increasing resistance to weight loss

Stage 2—Early Insulin Resistance
- Low HDL cholesterol
- Increasing Triglyceride levels
- Significant weight gain (central)—increasing waist size
- Increasing fatigue following a high-glycemic meal or snack
- Pattern of nighttime eating
- Increasing carbohydrate cravings, uncontrollable hunger, and emotional eating
- Menstrual irregularities
- Hypoglycemia
- Carbohydrate addiction—cravings for sugar and high-glycemic carbohydrates

Stage 3—Full-blown Insulin Resistance

(A patient must have 3 or more of the following 5 criteria to be diagnosed with the Metabolic Syndrome*)

- High blood pressure: >130/85 mm Hg
- Central Obesity: Waist size > than 34.5 inches (88 cm) in women; or > than 40 inches (102 cm) in men
- Elevated triglyceride level > the 150 (1.69 mmol/L)
- Low HDL cholesterol level: women < 50 mg/dl (1.29 mmol/L); men < 40 (1.04 mmol/L)
- Fasting glucose (blood sugar): > 110 mg/dL (>6.1 mmol/L)

Stage 4—Diabetes Mellitus (Type 2)

Patient has developed type 2 diabetes mellitus: Fasting blood sugar > 125 mg/dL (6.9 mmol/L)

*National Cholesterol Education Program Expert Panel Criteria for the Diagnosis of the Metabolic Syndrome.

WHAT COMES FIRST—OBESITY OR DIABETES?

One of the major debates in the medical community today is whether becoming overweight causes insulin insensitivity or the reverse—insulin resistance causes obesity. I am going to weigh in heavily on this argument (no pun intended) because it is key in understanding why you can't lose weight.

The media and medical community keep telling us the reason we are seeing an epidemic of type 2 diabetes mellitus is that more and more people are getting fatter. However, what has become very apparent to me after researching the medical literature and observing patients in my own clinical practice is that people are not only becoming overweight because of insulin resistance, but they are also developing type 2 diabetes mellitus because of insulin resistance.

The reason that this becomes so important is because physicians continue to tell their patients that they just need to lose some weight if they want to avoid becoming diabetic. However, one of the hallmark signs of insulin resistance is an inability to lose weight no matter what you try. This leads to a tremendous amount of frustration among patients because by the time they have seen the doctor and have been told that they are on the verge of becoming diabetic they have tried almost everything to lose weight without success. I have learned that unless these individuals reverse their underlying insulin resistance, they not only are not able to lose weight but they are also not able to prevent developing diabetes.

The epidemics of obesity and type 2 diabetes are the result of millions of people who are slowly entering the progression toward the metabolic syndrome. This fact becomes crucial in our approach to slowing down and even reversing both the increasing incidence of obesity and type 2 diabetes mellitus. It actually becomes the central answer to the obesity and diabetes epidemics that are undermining our health and threatening to bankrupt our health care system.

Critical to understanding that one of the primary consequences of insulin resistance is *central obesity is to look at the changes that occur when you first "tip over" into insulin resistance.* We then begin to understand why the medical community is referring to this metabolically active fat as "Killer Fat."

CENTRAL OBESITY OR KILLER FAT

Most of the serious weight gain, when it comes to our health, is central obesity (apple shaped). When we begin to gain weight around our middle, the adipose cells (fat cells) do not increase in number but rather increase in size. This means they simply become larger and larger until they are almost ready to burst. This is the type of weight gain that develops when you become insulin resistant. Because this weight gain is associated with all of these other metabolic changes like high blood pressure, abnormal elevation of lipids, heart disease, chronic inflammation, and diabetes, the medical community is now beginning to refer to centralized fat as, "Killer Fat."

Waist Size

Detecting whether or not you are developing central obesity is easy. Many physicians and researchers are now saying that patients only need to measure their waists. Dr. Jean-Pierre Despré's argues in favor of this method, "The waist circumference is a good index of the *absolute* amount of abdominal fat, whereas the waist to hip ratio (WHR) more adequately reflects *relative* abdominal deposition, which may not always be associated with high absolute levels of abdominal fat."

Researchers have determined that if a woman's waist size (circumference) is 34.5 inches (88cm) or greater, or a man's waist size is greater than 40 inches (102 cm), he or she has significant abdominal fat and is in danger. I actually become concerned when the women in my office present with a waist size greater than 30 inches and my men with a waist size greater than 36 inches. The measuring method doesn't have to be too fancy. Simply take a measuring tape and check your waist size. The best measurement is obtained by measuring about one inch below the belly button (umbilicus) and across the top to the pelvis (iliac crest).

As you learned earlier, insulin resistance and the metabolic syndrome takes years to develop. In other words, you don't develop the metabolic syndrome overnight and as a physician, I become concerned when I see a patient who suddenly begins to gain added inches around his or her waist. The waist measurement is one I now take during each and every physical exam I give. It is much more important than weight, height, body mass index, or the waist to hip ratio because of the serious health consequences involved or associated with central weight gain.

WHAT CAUSES THIS CENTRAL WEIGHT GAIN?

There is a switch that occurs mysteriously inside our bodies, which explains the unusual amount of central weight gain that occurs in patients who have just developed insulin resistance. Normally, 85 to 90% of all the glucose produced after eating a meal goes to the muscle cells to be either utilized for energy or stored as glycogen for immediate energy reserve in the muscle. This means that only 10 to 15% of the glucose ends up in our fat cells. If the insulin and glucagon levels are normal, there is a nice balance of fat being produced and broken down, and no weight gain occurs.

Animal studies reveal that when insulin resistance first develops, the muscle cells become insulin resistant first, before the fat cells do. This finding is critical because it means that the muscle is not able to utilize all the glucose it normally would following any meal or snack, and instead, a significant amount of that glucose is redirected to the fat cells of our abdomen.

As you learned earlier, when you first become insulin resistant the body compensates by making more and more insulin. Remember, insulin is our "fat storage hormone," and one of its jobs is to change sugar into fat. Since, in a normal setting, most of the glucose goes to the muscle cells, relatively little sugar remains available to be changed into fat. But when insulin resistance begins it is like someone or something mysteriously switches the tracks of your glucose train and a significant amount of sugar is now redirected from our muscles to the fat cells of our abdomen. Picture the blood sugar traveling around in a boxcar following the locomotive engine headed for your muscle cells. Then all of a sudden, early in the onset of insulin resistance, the tracks get switched and that train is diverted and heads straight for the storage bins—the fat cells of your abdomen.

This is a "one—two punch" that floors most of us. Insulin resistance not only increases the amount of insulin (our storage hormone) in our blood stream but our muscle cells are the first to become insulin resistant. Therefore, you are now diverting a significant amount of the glucose from a meal or snack to the fat cells of our abdomen. We then start gaining more and more weight in our waistlines even when there has not been a significant change in our diets or activity levels.

It may have taken years of abusing one's insulin with a high-glycemic diet and inactivity to get to this point, but when it happens, it always comes as a shock. One's waist measurement therefore must be a major consideration when determining whether or not he or she is developing insulin resistance and the resultant Killer Fat.

GETTING FATTER AND FATTER

As this process progresses, fat cells around our middle simply keep getting fatter and fatter. Each abdominal fat cell then begins to function poorly. They will eventually become resistant to insulin and begin releasing some of the fat they've been holding on to so tightly. This may seem like a good thing if you are trying to lose weight, but let me assure you it is not. First of all, fat will again be added at approximately the same rate as it is being released from the fat cells. However at this point, the abdominal fat cells begin releasing a large amount of fat into the blood stream in the form of triglycerides. This puts tremendous stress on both the beta cells of the pancreas (lipotoxicity) and obviously on the arteries. Individuals who have developed central obesity have been found to have significantly increased amounts of inflammation in their arteries. This serious condition is why physicians are beginning to refer to abdominal fat cells as being metabolically active and harmful to our health.

THE FALLACY OF A CALORIE IN AND A CALORIE OUT

You should be starting to realize a very important truth—when insulin resistance is involved, a calorie is not merely a calorie anymore. The fact is, your fat cells start acting like a sponge and soak up all the glucose and efficiently change it into fat no matter how many calories you try to burn. The concept of "a calorie in must equal a calorie out," which has been the mainstay of weight loss therapy throughout the past century needs to change. When you begin to recognize the affect that insulin resistance throws into this equation, a calorie is no longer just a calorie.

So many of my patients have come to me over the years complaining that they have mysteriously begun to gain weight in spite of the fact that they have not changed their eating habits or their activity level. My standard response used to be that I believed their metabolism had slowed down. I am sure you may have even heard similar comments from your physician. However, I now realize that the majority of the time, this mysterious weight gain is the result of the patient having "switched tracks." The individual who has just developed insulin resistance after years of abusing his or her insulin, will now gain an unusual amount of weight around their middle because they have now "tipped over" into this abnormal metabolic state. There has generally been no change in their eating habits or activity level; however, they now have developed a major weight problem. In fact, one of the hallmark signs of developing insulin resistance is the inability to lose weight. When you consider that nearly 50% of the adult population has some stage of insulin resistance, you can see why insulin resistance is a major aspect of our present obesity epidemic. **Until they reverse their underlying insulin resistance, they will not able to lose this weight no matter how hard they try!**

RELEASING FAT

After years and years of abusing your insulin by consuming tremendous amounts of high-glycemic carbohydrates day in and day out, you too are most likely becoming resistant to your insulin. A calorie is no longer a calorie because the tracks of this glucose train have been switched and your body is not functioning properly. If you don't learn how to switch the tracks back, you simply will not be able to lose weight even with the most aggressive diets. In this state, the body is resistant to almost any weight loss program.

Over the past twelve years of helping my patients develop healthy lifestyles, which corrects this underlying insulin resistance, I have witnessed an amazing phenomenon—my patients begin "releasing fat" and they are not even trying. My patients are amazed when they begin to realize the fat is simply melting away. They are not hungry (they are not restricting their calories) because they have had victory over their carbohydrate addiction. They are exercising consistently and providing their body with cellular nutrition. The weight loss they experience cannot be explained by a low-calorie (calories in) diet or by aggressive exercise (calories out). They just begin releasing fat as mysteriously as they had previously put it on. When I re-evaluate their blood work, I am able to note that their triglyceride/HDL cholesterol ratio has fallen below 2. This means that they have been able to reverse their insulin resistance and "tip back" into a normal metabolic state. They have literally switched the tracks of their glucose train back to their muscle.

If you are not able to lose weight, it's not because one day your fat burning ability disappeared. If your doctor has told you that the reason you have begun putting on weight because your metabolism has declined, he or she is mistaken in the overwhelming majority of cases. The truth is, the tracks of your glucose train have been switched and a significant amount of glucose is now being delivered to the fat cells of your abdomen to be stored as fat rather than to your muscles to be utilized for energy. The only answer to this dilemma is a program designed to reverse insulin resistance and allow you to successfully "flip the switch back again." That is what this booklet and the Healthy for Life Program is all about. We now need to focus on exactly what you can do to prevent or reverse this underlying insulin resistance and allow you to not only prevent becoming diabetic but also allow you to lose weight permanently.

PART 2

PREVENTING OR REVERSING INSULIN RESISTANCE

The goal of this booklet is to show you how you can take control of your own health and literally prevent ever developing diabetes. If you have already developed diabetes, it will show you how you can best control or even possibly even reverse your diabetes. People falsely believe that they have no choice in whether or not they develop diabetes. They believe it is just in the cards they have been dealt. Maybe one or both of their parents were diabetic and it is just in their genes. Genetics are part of the problem; however, even if you are genetically predisposed to developing diabetes, establishing these healthy lifestyles will give you the absolute best chance of avoiding ever becoming diabetic. Truly, you are in control and the decisions you make and the lifestyles you choose from this day forward will determine the health problems you most likely will encounter. Is it worth it? Life passes us by very fast. Why make it faster by falling into the trap of insulin resistance?

How difficult is it to make these changes? Well, you will never have to go hungry, you will have more energy, more focus, your health parameters will improve, and—by the way—you will have permanent weight loss. Remember, the Healthy for Life Program is NOT a diet. It is a lifestyle. These are lifestyle changes you need to be making for the rest of your life.

HEALTHY FOR LIFE PROGRAM

Throughout this booklet, I have presented cutting-edge medical and scientific information; however it is very important that this knowledge become practical and useful to you. Thirty years of private family practice has taught me that I must keep instructions simple and doable. Being practical is imperative in allowing my patients to achieve the success and goals they desire. This booklet will provide the basic instructions of the Healthy for Life Program. If you would like more detailed information, I would encourage you to pick up a copy of my book *Releasing Fat*. Better yet, check out my interactive web page at **www.releasingfat.com**. Take the "free" automated health risk assessment and learn where you stand in regards to insulin resistance in your own life. Take the web site tour and check out the overview to this remarkable Internet behavioral modification program. These tools will give you the best opportunity to personally change your health destiny for a lifetime. Remember, the answers you seek cannot be found in the medication I prescribe, but rather in your daily lifestyle choices.

FIRST-STEP THERAPY

It is a well-known fact that the majority of the top ten leading causes of death in the modern world today are the result of our lifestyle. Heart attacks, cancer, strokes, diabetes, hypertension, obesity, and osteoporosis are some of the major diseases that are directly related to our unhealthy lifestyles. This is why physicians are encouraged to allow their patients a trial of improved lifestyles before they begin treating any of these diseases with drugs. When I initially diagnose a patient with diabetes, I always try to offer my patients a chance to improve their lifestyles whenever possible as a means of controlling their diabetes. Hopefully they won't even have to begin medication. In the medical community, this is called first-step therapy. However, today most physicians simply give this recommendation lip service and begin their patients on medication before they have had a trial of these healthy lifestyle changes. I personally believe that this has happened because most physicians wrongly assume that their patients will not successfully make these healthy lifestyle changes. Others believe that even if they make lifestyle changes that they will not be effective in improving their clinical problem.

Over the past ten years, I have realized some very important truths. First, the majority of my patients (over 80% in my clinical experience) would rather make healthy lifestyle changes than begin taking medication. Even if there is the slightest chance of avoiding a drug, the patient desires to make these healthy lifestyle changes first. Second, I have learned that when the triad of healthy lifestyles recommended in the Healthy for Life Program are implemented, most people are able to improve clinically and avoid the need for medication altogether. The reason is really quite simple: the underlying cause of the medical problem in the majority of cases is actually corrected, which is insulin resistance.

If you are personally facing the prospect of needing medication or desiring to get off medication that has already been started, the Healthy for Life Program may be just what you need. Let me make one thing very clear; however, *you must remain under the direct supervision of your personal physician.* No one (and I mean no one!) should discontinue any medication prescribed by a physician without his or her doctor's direction and permission. If you are already taking medication, you should only come off that medication after your physician has documented positive clinical results from your healthy lifestyle changes. In most cases, this may take several months to one or two years to accomplish. I have found that most physicians are willing to work closely with their patient when the patient strongly desires to avoid starting a medication or is trying to get off a prescription. In fact, more and more physicians are recommending the Healthy for Life Internet Program to their patients and it has become their wellness program.

Another warning is the fact that diabetics will generally see significant improvement in their blood sugars and their diabetic control the longer they are involved in the program. Some even note dramatic improvement within the first few weeks. If you are diabetic and on medication or insulin, you must be checking your blood sugars at least 4 times daily during the first few weeks of the program. If your blood sugars begin to drop and fall into the low blood sugar range (hypoglycemic range), contact your physician immediately so that he or she can readjust your medication. Also, do not worry if your blood sugars go up a little initially. Remember, the mere fact that you are already diabetic means that you are further down the line in regards to having significant insulin resistance. It usually takes my diabetic patients 18 to 24 months on this program before they have received the full potential value from these healthy lifestyles.

TRIAD OF HEALTHY LIFESTYLES

The success of this program is the result of a healthy diet that does not spike one's blood sugar, developing a moderate, consistent exercise program, and taking high-quality nutritional supplements that provide cellular nutrition. I am sure you may have tried different aspects of the program before in other settings. You may have tried a similar diet program or had a great exercise program or maybe you even taken optimal levels of high-quality nutritional supplements and still have not had lasting success. Let me tell you why. **The secret lies in the combination of all three of these healthy lifestyles that are implemented together in a carefully balanced fashion.**

Over the past twelve years, I have worked with hundreds of patients who have had tremendous results in preventing, controlling, and even reversing their diabetes. However, I have learned one unmistakable principle during this same period of time: if my patients will make one of these lifestyle changes, they definitely do better. It does not matter if they begin eating healthy or start an exercise program or begin by taking high-quality nutritional supplements. They will have some success. If they make two of the three lifestyle changes, they do even a little better. However, when they are willing to embrace all three of these changes together, the results are simply amazing.

You must remember that insulin resistance is a very difficult disease process to actually reverse. You have been developing this problem for decades and it is not going to reverse overnight. However, the body has an amazing ability to heal itself. Every aspect of the Healthy for Life Program actually improves insulin sensitivity in a different manner. When you combine all three aspects of the Healthy for Life Program together, you give yourself the absolute best chance of reversing this underlying insulin resistance and achieving your health goals. But remember, it takes time to firmly establish these new, healthier lifestyles and time for these lifestyles to reverse the consequences of years of unhealthy lifestyles.

DR. RAY STRAND, M.D.

HEALTHY DIET
Carbohydrates

When I say the word, "carbohydrate," what comes to your mind? Most people think of starches: bread, potatoes, rice, and crackers. Why? Because we've been taught since elementary school that complex carbohydrates such as these are the healthiest choices. After all they make up the broadest portion of the USDA food pyramid, right? It has long been believed that these foods break down into glucose more slowly, thus providing a continual release of energy to the body, making them the best choice. However, this theory is now being seriously challenged and I believe we may have finally discovered the missing link to our nation's obesity mystery.

SIMPLE OR COMPLEX?

One thing is for certain: carbohydrates are not equal. We cannot exchange one calorie for another as infamous diet programs and diets taught our diabetic patients have been teaching all along. Carbohydrates are simply long chains of sugars. Digestion rate, and thus the rise in blood sugar after eating a particular carbohydrate, has commonly been believed to be determined by the length of the sugar chain. Shorter chains were considered simple carbohydrates and longer chains, complex.

The concept of simple sugar versus complex carbohydrates was first introduced in 1901 and has prevailed throughout the entire 20th century and now into the 21st century. Since the inception of this theory, scientists have held rigidly to the belief that if you eat a simple sugar like glucose, fructose, maltose, or sucrose your blood sugar would rise rapidly because your body does not need to break down the sugar. However; if you eat a complex carbohydrate with longer chains of sugars, like a potato or a piece of bread, your blood sugar would rise more slowly and therefore would be a better choice for diabetics. This is why you see grains and breads on the bottom rung of the food pyramid (even the new revised USDA food pyramid) and simple sugars such as candy and sweets at its peak.

Because this concept of simple and complex carbohydrates has been the standard of care for the medical community for well over 100 years it has become firmly imbedded in our thinking and our practice of medicine. In fact, this underlying theory is still primarily taught to our diabetics in the US. It's hard to change a concept that has been with us for so long. However, I believe this fallacy is the main reason our diabetics are doing so poorly and that we are facing such an overwhelming health care crisis in the United States and around the world.

As the concept of a low-fat, high-carbohydrate diet gained acceptance in the early 1970's, the basic recommendation was that any carbohydrate other than sugar was acceptable in newly recommended "healthy" diets. While no distinction was made between the different characteristics of complex carbohydrates, the focus was primarily on teaching our nation to decrease the amount of fat being consumed in one's diet.

A Revolutionary Breakthrough—the Glycemic Index

The glycemic index is simply a numerical system that rates how fast carbohydrates break down into glucose and enter the bloodstream. This concept has radically changed the way we look at carbohydrates. Instead of accepting the theory that the rate of absorption and thus the rise of blood sugar is simply based on the length of the chain and complexity of the sugar being consumed, the actual rise in the blood sugar is now being determined in a clinical setting with standardized techniques.

It wasn't until 1981, that a researcher by the name of Dr. David Jenkins introduced this new concept in the *American Journal of Clinical Nutrition*. Dr. Jenkins defined the glycemic index as the rate blood sugar rises following the ingestion of a particular test food relative to that of a standard food (usually white bread or glucose). All other carbohydrates are then compared to glucose, which was given a glycemic index of 100. See table 2 to get an idea of the glycemic index of some common foods.

TABLE 2
Glycemic Index and Glycemic Load of Some Common Foods

	GLYCEMIC INDEX	CARBOHYDRATES PER SERVING	GLYCEMIC LOAD
Glucose	100	10	10
Fructose (fruit sugar)	19	10	6
Sucrose (table sugar)	61	10	6
Bakery Goods			
Angel Food Cake	67	29	19
Croissant	67	26	17
Doughnut, cake	76	23	17
Muffin, bran	60	24	15
Vegetables			
Carrots	47	6	3
Peas	48	7	3
Corn, sweet	54	17	9
Fruits			
Apple	38	16	6
Cherries	22	12	3
Orange	42	11	5
Peach	28	13	4

	GLYCEMIC INDEX	CARBOHYDRATES PER SERVING	GLYCEMIC LOAD
Legumes			
Beans, kidney	28	25	7
Beans, black	20	25	5
Breads			
Bagel, white	72	35	25
Bread, white	70	14	10
Bread, whole-wheat flour	71	16	8
Potato			
Baked, white	85	30	26
Instant, mashed	85	20	17
Mashed Potato	92	20	18

When the glycemic index was first released, most dieticians, nutritionists, and physicians were shocked by the results. Why? It flew in the face of the theory that all carbohydrates are created equal. For example, simple sugars like table sugar (sucrose) had a glycemic index of 61 while the sugar found in fruits (fructose) had a glycemic index of only 19.

What were we to do with our food pyramid upon discovering the score of complex carbohydrates such as white potatoes (glycemic index of 85), or white bread (in the 70 range) making both these foods spike blood sugar more readily than table sugar? Did you know that many of our "healthy" breakfast cereals such as corn flakes, bran flakes, and Cheerios top out the glycemic index, some scoring as high as 92?!

These findings literally shot down the concept that the rise in blood sugar can be determined solely on the premise of whether a carbohydrate is a simple sugar or a complex carbohydrate. I'd say we can definitely anticipate some resistance to such shocking scores because it means our medical professionals have been advising diabetics to eat carbohydrates that can dangerously spike their blood sugars. When I am consulting new diabetic patients in my office to these truths and concepts, they almost universally tell me that they already know that these foods spike their blood sugars because they have checked their blood sugars after eating these types of foods. They essentially have lost all confidence in the medical community because of the diet that their doctor and dieticians have been recommending they eat.

There is no doubt in my mind that after adequately reviewing the medical literature regarding the glycemic index, America will soon follow and accept this scientific standard. In fact, in the May 8, 2002 issue of the *Journal of the American Medical Association,* an article was presented wherein a review was made of 311 studies dealing with the glycemic index. Studies and reports such as these will undoubtedly impact the medical community and bring about much needed change.

Why should those of us who have diabetes or even don't have diabetes be concerned about the glycemic index? Since we are now realizing that simple sugars and complex carbohydrates no longer give us any indication of how fast our bodies will absorb the foods we eat, we must know what *does* determine our body's ability to absorb a particular food so we can wisely choose foods that don't spike our blood sugar. The most dangerous blood sugar for the diabetic is not the fasting blood sugar, but instead, their blood sugar level following a meal or snack. This is called the postprandial blood sugar and it is defined as the level of blood sugar obtained one to two hours after eating a meal or snack. Medical research is now showing us that this is the time that those who have diabetes or insulin resistance should be concerned because this is when most of the damage is occurring to our arteries. This is the result of the glycemic stress we talked about earlier.

The discovery of the glycemic index has allowed us to realize that our bodies are able to absorb the glucose from these high-glycemic foods very quickly. This results in a rapid rise of our blood sugar and creates tremendous inflammation and spasm of our arteries. In fact, studies have shown that when you spike your blood sugar that your arteries literally go into spasm for 3 to 4 hours after that meal. Not only does it lead to insulin resistance, but it also is the main reason diabetics' arteries age so fast.

Think for a moment about the number of processed grains and carbohydrates that are in our diet: white breads and pastries, pizza crust, hamburger buns, most rice, pasta, crackers, cakes, cookies, donuts, and breakfast cereals. Now take a look at the glycemic index of some fruits, vegetables and legumes listed in Table 2.

EVENTS FOLLOWING A HIGH-GLYCEMIC MEAL—A REVIEW

Following a breakfast of instant oatmeal, white toast, and sweetened orange juice our blood sugar begins to rise rapidly. This spike in blood sugar, as you know, will almost immediately stimulate a heavy release of insulin and in turn significantly suppress the release of glucagon. Glucagon is a hormone that has the opposite affect of insulin in the body. It is our "fat releasing" hormone. The high levels of insulin now drive the sugar into the muscle, liver, and fat to be either utilized or stored as glycogen or fat. Because of this excessive release of insulin our blood sugar begins to fall almost as rapidly as it climbed. In fact, it will usually fall well below the fasting blood sugar level into what is known as a "hypoglycemic range" (low blood sugar). See Figure 1

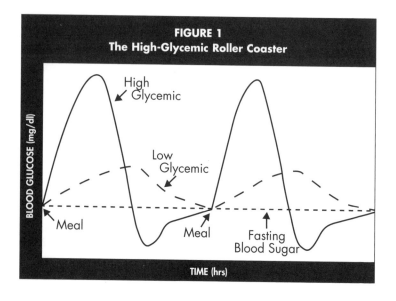

FIGURE 1
The High-Glycemic Roller Coaster

The body must control blood sugar in a very narrow range primarily because the brain thinks by using blood sugar as its number one fuel source. If the blood sugar is allowed to continue to fall, you not only can have a shaky weakness and become mentally confused, but you can also have a seizure or go into a coma. Because the body needs to bring this blood sugar up, this low blood sugar stimulates the release of what are known as the stress hormones like cortisol and adrenaline. These stress hormones' primary purpose is to get the blood sugar back up to acceptable levels. Although the blood sugar eventually does return to normal you now have high levels of stress hormones floating around in your blood stream. This leaves you with what I refer to as an "uncontrollable hunger" and you have to eat again—you have no choice. Typically at this point you will crave another high-glycemic snack or meal and this cycle is repeated again. This state of uncontrollable hunger may stay with you for several hours to even a day or two after spiking your blood sugar just one time. So not only does spiking your blood sugar cause inflammation and damage to your arteries, but it also leads to this uncontrollable hunger and what I refer to as a carbohydrate addiction.

What you have always considered emotional eating or cravings are really just this natural physiological response to these low blood sugars. You really have no choice—you must eat again. It is like trying to avoid using the restroom when your body is signaling that your bladder is full. You may smile a lot and cross your legs tightly; however, if you do not give into the warning signs, *you will go* whether or not you're in the restroom! A similar physiological response takes place when you experience a feeling of uncontrollable hunger. You may fight it for a while, but in the end you have to give in and eat something. Call it hunger, a craving, emotional eating, or an addiction; in the end, it leads to your downfall and forces you to do exactly the opposite of what you desire to do in the first place—eat less food.

To illustrate the powerful difference between high- and low-glycemic carbohydrates, young boys were given either a high-glycemic breakfast or a low-glycemic breakfast that contained the same amount of calories. They were then given either a low-glycemic or high-glycemic lunch of equal calories. Following the noon meal, the boys were allowed to eat anything they desired for the rest of the day. What the researchers observed was that the boys who ate the high-glycemic meals ate over 80% more calories than the boys who ate the low-glycemic meals. Just to make sure there wasn't any difference in the two groups, the researchers switched the meals between the two groups of boys and again found that the boys who ate the high-glycemic meals ate 80% more calories than the boys who ate the low-glycemic meals. This study clearly illustrates the trap so many of us find ourselves. It is truly a vicious cycle that I have labeled a "carbohydrate addiction".

CARBOHYDRATE ADDICTION

Americans are one of the largest groups of carbohydrate addicts. Unknowingly, we have become addicted to processed carbohydrates much like people became addicted to cigarettes years ago. We keep spiking our blood sugar, which quickly drops because of the over stimulation of insulin. This leads to the uncontrollable craving for another high-glycemic meal and we not only overeat, but also continue this vicious cycle.

The rush of a roller coaster ride is fun once a year or so, but it wouldn't be good if we continued riding day after day for decades at a time. The rapid rise and fall of our blood sugar is more dangerous still. Not only does eating the typical American diet cause us to store more fat, we literally become hooked—on processed and high-glycemic carbohydrates. And just like a chain smoker aches for nicotine, our cravings make us go back for more and more empty calories. Soon the abuse of insulin turns into an addiction and the addiction takes over the controls. We are no longer free to choose. We are driven to high-glycemic carbohydrates. If you don't think so, just see how ugly it gets when someone suggests that you need to replace your favorite snacks with healthy carbohydrates!

If you look at Figure 1 again, you can see why you may feel good for 20 to 30 minutes after a bag of snack crackers and a soda. It's because your blood sugar is peaking, but in just minutes it will come crashing down again. And since your brain operates on blood sugar, it is going to do everything it can to get you to eat more so you can raise this blood sugar again. This is the main reason so many people fail with dieting.

You may be trying to eat less food to lower your caloric intake only to find that you have a relentless craving for more. After gorging yourself full of whatever you can find, you then become discouraged because you believe your will power is not strong enough. In reality, you are being set up for failure by the body's natural response to high-glycemic carbohydrate diets.

We can therefore, deduce with accuracy that the low-fat, high-carbohydrate (primarily highly processed, high-glycemic) diet that you have been faithfully trying to follow all of these years, is actually doing you more harm than good. You end up eating more calories, gaining more weight, and losing your health all at the same time.

GRAMS OF CARBOHYDRATES

At this point it is very important to caution those of you who are involved with the low-carbohydrate craze and are into counting grams of carbohydrates. One of the most popular diets today is the Atkin's diet. Now many diabetics have learned that carbohydrates are bad for them and that they need to be avoided altogether. They actually begin to panic when anyone even suggests that they should begin eating more carbohydrates. They focus on the amount or grams of carbohydrates a particular food or meal contain and don't take into consideration the glycemic index. The body needs and desires carbohydrates. These are the foods that contain all of those good vitamins, minerals, and antioxidants the body needs and desires. Foods like whole fruits, vegetables, and whole grains are critical for our health—even the health of the diabetic. You need to remember that there are good carbohydrates and there are bad carbohydrates. You want to be consuming those good carbohydrates that do not spike your blood sugar. However, another critical aspect in choosing those good, healthy carbohydrates is understanding the concept of glycemic load. To learn more about which carbohydrates are desirable get a copy of my book, Releasing Fat (Health Concepts 2004) or join my Healthy for Life Program at www.releasingfat.com.

CONCEPT OF GLYCEMIC LOAD

Since the concept of glycemic index is relatively new to most people, there is often some confusion about how exactly to interpret its practical use as a guide to healthy nutrition. One of the major reasons we'll want to become familiar with the glycemic index of most common foods is to avoid the problem of spiking our blood sugar and subsequently our blood insulin levels following a meal. In order to better understand its use, we need to understand the concept of glycemic load.

Glycemic load is defined as the weighted average glycemic index of an individual food multiplied by the percentage of dietary energy (grams of carbohydrates or calories) contained. A simple calculation allows you to arrive at the glycemic load of any food. You can usually locate the grams of carbohydrate in a particular food and then multiplying it by the glycemic index. Then you divide this number by 100.

The concept of glycemic load provides a much better picture of one's response to a particular food. For example, cooked carrots have a medium glycemic index of 49 while its glycemic load is 2.4

(because there are very few calories in carrots). This means that eating carrots cannot spike your blood sugar. However, potatoes have both a high glycemic index and a high glycemic load, which will significantly raise the blood sugar and stimulate a heightened insulin response.

Determining the Glycemic Load

Glycemic load= (Glycemic Index x Grams of Carbohydrate) divided by 100

Spaghetti: 1 cup of cooked spaghetti has a Glycemic Index of 41 and contains 52 grams of carbohydrate.

Glycemic Load: (41x52) divided by 100 = 21

Carrots: Glycemic index is 49 and the average serving contains an average of 5 grams of carbohydrates per serving.

Glycemic Load: (49 x 5) divided by 100 = 2.4

This example illustrates the fact that the glycemic index is only one aspect in choosing quality carbohydrates. If you were to only consider the glycemic index, spaghetti looks like a better choice than carrots. However, when you look at the grams of carbohydrates you are consuming with one serving (2 ounces or $1/2$ cup) of spaghetti (52 grams) compared with the amount of carbohydrates consumed with an average serving of carrots (5 grams), it becomes apparent that the spaghetti is going to create a greater rise in our blood sugar and insulin response, especially when you consider few of us eat just one-half cup of spaghetti for an average serving.

DETERMINING THE GLYCEMIC INDEX
OF MIXED MEALS

One of the major arguments against using the glycemic index for clinical studies stems from the theory that when carbohydrates, fats, and proteins are mixed together into a regular meal, all carbohydrates are absorbed at the same rate. Initially, there were a few studies that supported this viewpoint. But, an overwhelming number of recent studies definitely support the fact that the glycemic index of various carbohydrates eaten during any particular meal closely correlate with the glycemic index of that meal.

Fats will slow gastric emptying (the rate at which food leaves the stomach to be absorbed by the small bowel) and therefore lowers the glycemic index of a mixed meal. In fact, this has become another major concern with the low-fat, high-carbohydrate diet. The fact remains that when individuals eat more carbohydrates in their diet, they also tend to eat less fat (including the necessary fats). This causes even greater spikes in their blood sugars following these meals. However, over the years, more and more studies show that when you consider the glycemic index of various foods in a particular meal, you are able to accurately predict the glycemic and insulin response to that meal and therefore make intentionally healthy choices.

A carbohydrate is not just a carbohydrate and one calorie cannot be exchanged for another. Until we are willing to take a good hard look at what we eat every day—in every meal and snack—our nation's severe health risks will continue to multiply.

Our society is reaping the health consequences of many addictions, one of them being tobacco. It's astounding to note, that one can become addicted to nicotine within the first week or two of trying cigarettes. We all realize now that smoking can lead to heart attacks, strokes, lung cancer, and emphysema. The health care costs are astronomical. However, we are just now beginning to realize that high-glycemic foods can be as addictive as smoking and are the major reason health consequences of obesity are now surpassing the health care costs of tobacco abuse.

Again, I want to warn every one of you at this point. Carbohydrates are NOT the enemy. I am not advocating a low- or no-carbohydrate diet. The body needs and desires carbohydrates. So it is critical that you do not focus on how many carbohydrates a particular food or meal may contain, but instead, become familiar with the glycemic index and glycemic load of the carbohydrates you are consuming. There are good carbohydrates and there are bad carbohydrates. Just like we learn there are good fats and there are bad fats. The good carbohydrates like whole fruits, whole vegetables, and whole grains contain those important vitamins, minerals, and antioxidants the body needs. These are low-glycemic and do not spike your blood sugar, which is critical for anyone who desires to prevent or control diabetes. It is important to realize what happens when you begin to eat these kinds of foods.

EVENTS FOLLOWING A LOW-GLYCEMIC MEAL

Compare what transpires when an individual eats a meal consisting of low-glycemic carbohydrates, instead of a high-glycemic meal. (Again, this means eating foods like whole fruits, whole vegetables, and whole grains along with some good protein and good fat. In this case, the blood sugar rises slowly; therefore, not over stimulating the release of insulin. The blood sugar comes down very slowly and you remain satisfied much longer following a meal like this. If you are diabetic, this is what you want to happen. If your blood sugar doesn't go shooting up, you don't have to take so much insulin or medication to bring it down. Plus, you must remember that the first hour or two following your meal is the most critical time for the diabetic. Now your blood sugar is also not going to fall into this low blood sugar range; therefore, you do not stimulate the release of these stress hormones and don't set off this uncontrollable hunger. [See Figure 1—and look at the broken line, which is the blood sugar response to a low-glycemic meal] Following a meal like this your blood insulin levels will begin to fall and glucagon levels begin to rise. Now let's look at what glucagon does in the body.

Glucagon is your fat releasing hormone. You need to be elevating your glucagon levels if you are going to have any hope of releasing fat. When you are addicted to high-glycemic carbohydrates, you are continually stimulating the release of insulin and suppressing the release of glucagon. When you begin to eat balanced, low-glycemic meals, you are going to be lowering your insulin levels and increasing your glucagon levels. The key to the Healthy for Life Program is allowing your glucagon levels to remain higher, which improves insulin resistance. This allows you to be able to reverse all the unhealthy consequences of your former lifestyle.

GOOD FATS

For nearly 40 years now we have heard little other than the harm that comes from consuming too much fat. Medical science has shown evidence that the higher your total cholesterol level and LDL (bad cholesterol), the greater is your risk of developing cardiovascular disease. As a result of all of the medical and media attention to the harmful aspects of fat in our diets, we've become fearful of fat. I don't believe there has been more misinformation on any other given topic during my thirty-year career as a clinician.

The truth is that not all fats are bad and to the contrary, fats are essential for our health. The body requires carbohydrates, proteins, *and fats* to survive. Fat is needed to build our cell membranes, brain cells, nerves, and many of our hormones. Fat is not the problem, but rather *the kinds* of fat we consume. The biochemistry behind the various fats in our body will help differentiate between a good fat and a bad fat.

When you consume monosaturated fat and the essential fatty acids (especially omega-3 fatty acids), you actually decrease your total cholesterol and LDL cholesterol. More importantly, good fat in a meal or snack also slows down gastric emptying. In other words, food remains in the stomach longer following a meal containing good fat, which means you will not absorb the nutrients from that meal as quickly. This is important because almost all of the absorption of the nutrients occurs in the small intestine. Therefore, blood sugars will tend to rise even slower when fat is included in your meal or snack.

Believe it or not, you need to eat good fat in order to lose fat. This statement goes against conventional wisdom from the last 40 years. The medical evidence now strongly supports this new position. The key is to consume good fats that actually decrease your total and LDL cholesterol levels while providing the fat the body needs to make healthy cell membranes, brain and nerve cells, and hormones. However, the key is to also be decreasing your consumption of the bad fats—saturated and trans-fats—while at the same time increasing your consumption of the good fats—monosaturated fats and omega-3 essential fatty acids. Fat consumption does not stimulate the release of either insulin or glucagon; however, because it slows down gastric emptying, it improves insulin resistance by not allowing the blood sugar to spike as high following a meal or a snack. Combining good fat with low-glycemic carbohydrates with your meal is a major step in allowing you to release fat. Now we need to look at the role of protein in your diet.

GOOD PROTEIN

Protein is essential for our existence. In fact, protein is more plentiful than any other substance in the body other than water. Our muscles, skin, hair, eyes, and nails are primarily made of protein. It is the main component of most of our enzymes and the cells that make up our immune system. All proteins are made from building blocks called amino acids. Protein is made up of twenty very important amino acids, ten of which are considered essential. This means that the body is unable to make these ten essential amino acid building blocks and if our bodies are going to survive they must be provided by our diets.

You may wonder why protein, if it is so important to our diet, is so maligned? Similar to fat, protein has been attacked almost as much and as consistently as fat. This, in part, may be due to the fact that the majority of protein eaten in this country comes from red meat and dairy products, and both are loaded with saturated fat.

Many nutritionists and researchers discredit vegetable proteins even though they contain less fat because they are incomplete and do not contain all of the ten essential amino acids. Protein deficiency is very rare in this country and many vegetarians have learned to utilize a variety of plant proteins, like beans, soy, lentils, and nuts to assure they are getting all the essential amino acids into their daily diet.

When you eat primarily plant protein you decrease your intake of saturated fat and decrease your exposure to toxic exposure (hormones, toxins, antibiotics) contained in meat and dairy products. However, vegetarians are not exempt from developing insulin resistance. If you are vegetarian or considering a vegetarian lifestyle, you also need to become conscientious about eliminating processed carbohydrates from your diet, since the average vegetarian is consuming 80% of his or her calories from carbohydrates. The frequency of insulin resistance is relatively high in vegetarians as it is with those that are meat lovers.

BEST SOURCES OF FAT AND PROTEIN

Best sources of fat/protein: Nuts, avocadoes, olives, beans, soy, and legumes

Second best sources of fat/protein: Cold-water fish like salmon, mackerel, trout, sardines, and some tuna (contains good quality protein and are high in omega-3 fatty acids).

Third best sources of fat/protein: Fowl even though this protein contains saturated fat, the fat of the bird is primarily on the outside of the meat and not marbled into the meat and can easily be removed.

Poorest sources of fat/protein: red meats, highly processed foods, and dairy products. When eating red meat purchase the leanest meat available. Choose from: wild game, buffalo, grass-fed cattle, organically raised cattle, turkey bacon, and turkey burgers.

HEALTHY FOR LIFE FOOD PYRAMID

Have you taken a look at the USDA food pyramid recently-even the new, revised one? It's fairly easy to find—you'll find it in children's textbooks and on the boxes of cereal and bread sacks. Do you know why? Bread and cereals have historically formed the broadest rung of the pyramid. Its primary focus is on decreasing the consumption of any kind of fat, while encouraging generous recommendations of grains and highly processed carbohydrates. The next question is who formulated the food pyramid? Like many health campaigns in this nation, the USDA food pyramid has been more politically motivated than based on science.

The Healthy for Life Food Pyramid, on the other hand, is science-based and is primarily focused on the consumption of good carbohydrates, good proteins, and good fats. When you look at this new pyramid [see Figure 2], you will see that the base is built with good carbohydrates such as: whole fruits and vegetables. You need to be eating eight to twelve servings of whole fruits and vegetables each and every day. This will most likely be the landmark change made to your choice in foods. You will need to reorganize the number and size of your food portions as well as your pantry. Eight to twelve servings may seem like too many, but keep in mind that many of our typical portions actually count for two or more servings.

Remember, carbohydrates are not the problem—*processed and high-glycemic carbohydrates* are. This change is the most critical aspect of the healthy lifestyles needed to reverse any of the stages of insulin resistance and allow you to release fat. Processed carbohydrates are your main enemy in achieving your goal of being able to reverse insulin resistance and begin releasing fat. However, eliminating or significantly decreasing all carbohydrates from your diet will create even greater health problems. Good carbohydrates are the main source of our vitamins, antioxidants, and minerals as well as the fuel source the body prefers (glucose).

Proteins and Fats make up the second level of the Healthy for Life Food Pyramid. The best protein is found in vegetables, legumes, and nuts. These proteins rate the highest because they

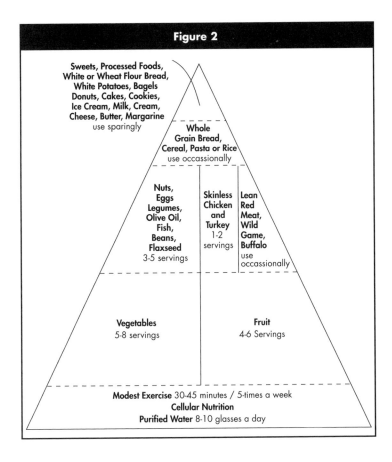

Figure 2

Sweets, Processed Foods,
White or Wheat Flour Bread,
White Potatoes, Bagels
Donuts, Cakes, Cookies,
Ice Cream, Milk, Cream,
Cheese, Butter, Margarine
use sparingly

Whole
Grain Bread,
Cereal, Pasta or Rice
use occassionally

Nuts,
Eggs
Legumes,
Olive Oil,
Fish,
Beans,
Flaxseed
3-5 servings

Skinless
Chicken
and
Turkey
1-2
servings

Lean
Red
Meat,
Wild
Game,
Buffalo
use
occassionally

Vegetables
5-8 servings

Fruit
4-6 Servings

Modest Exercise 30-45 minutes / 5-times a week
Cellular Nutrition
Purified Water 8-10 glasses a day

also contain all of the good fats (omega-3 and monosaturated fats). These foods also contain the phytochemicals and micronutrients your body needs as well as fewer toxins than animal fats. These foods are also low-glycemic foods. The next best protein comes from cold-water fish, which contain high levels of the omega-3 essential fats. The third best source of protein comes from foul, wild game, lean pork, and lean red meats.

Whole grains and whole cereals make up the third level of your new food pyramid. These are not processed carbohydrates, rather, whole rolled-oats, whole wheat, steel-cut oats, barley, whole wheat bread, etc. I have placed them at this level because overall we need to cut down our quantity of these carbs. When we consume these foods, it is critical that they are made from whole grains and not white or wheat flour.

The top of the food pyramid is made up of all the sweets, pastries, cakes, donuts, white bread, white flour, processed rice, bagels, etc. This is logical since all of these particular foods spike the blood sugar more quickly than even table sugar or candy. These must all be treated like candy.

Proper Balance between Carbohydrates, Fats, and Proteins

The balance with which you consume the three major macronutrients: carbohydrates, proteins, and fats, has been the subject of debate among many of the leading weight loss experts and health care professionals for years. I generally recommend that between 40 to 50 percent of your calories come from carbohydrates, 25 to 30 percent of your calories come from fat and 20 to 25 percent of your calories come from protein. Changing the balance of these macronutrients has been the driving theory behind the work of Dr. Dean Ornish, Dr. Robert Atkins, and Dr. Barry Sears for the past 30 years. The health care community also has its diet recommendations published through the American Heart Association, the American Diabetes Association, and the US Health Department. Needless-to-say, dietary advice often leaves consumers confused and uncertain as to what is best.

Obviously, since over one-third of the population is presently trying to lose weight and another third is trying to maintain their weight, losing weight is typically the leading consideration in determining which diet is chosen. Be assured, the Healthy for Life Program will not only allow you to lose fat effectively but it will also be a healthy diet that is not affected by politics, hype, or popular trends.

The most important key to this eating plan is not necessarily the balance between these nutrients; rather its focus is on the quality of the individual carbohydrates, proteins, and fats you choose to eat. The goal of a healthy eating plan is to eat the foods that provide the body with necessary building blocks to make healthy cells, enhance the body's natural antioxidant defense system, natural immune system, natural repair system, while providing hormonal balance. Your body not only needs a healthy balance between these macronutrients; it also requires *high quality* carbohydrates, fats, and proteins.

No Calorie Counting or Food Restriction

There has been an overriding concept in the medical community and weight loss industry over the past decade—the calories in need to be less than calories out. This philosophy maintains that in order to lose weight you need to take in fewer calories than your body utilizes. This has ushered in the low-calorie to *very* low-calorie diets that permeate the weight loss market today. Quick weight loss is the order of the day and this is primarily achieved by recommending diet plans that contain a significant restriction in the amount of calories you can consume. This leaves the participants in these diet plans hungry most of the time and their will power is challenged every hour of the day. Experience has shown us that individuals do not (cannot!) stay on these diets for any length of time and that the weight they do lose quickly returns. In contrast, there is no food restriction or calorie counting in my Healthy for

Life Program. This is a bold move for any program that is being developed not only to improve health but also to create fat loss for those who need to lose weight. If you don't need to lose weight, but are instead primarily concerned about improving control of your diabetes, then you will not lose weight. Since there is no calorie restriction with this program, you merely have to consume enough of all these good foods to maintain your weight. Your blood sugars and diabetic control will still improve.

The medical literature reveals that when children and adults are educated in what needs to be eaten for an ongoing healthy diet, they lose their fat even when they are not restricting their calories. Obviously, individuals will stay with a healthy eating plan that allows them to eat whenever they choose. When you eat a diet that does not spike your blood sugar, your insulin to glucagon ratio is excellent and your body functions the way it needs and wants to function. These meals and snacks create significant and prolonged satisfaction and when your hunger returns, you simply need to eat another low-glycemic meal or snack.

It is freeing to realize that when you eat correctly you will not experience the tremendous cravings and hunger you may have experienced with traditional weight loss programs. Also, you feel energetic, focused, and able to function at your optimal level because you are providing the fuel the body desires to use (glucose) at the appropriate levels. This is in contrast to the uncomfortable, fatigued feeling you have when you are using secondary fuel sources (like ketones) that are created with very low-carb diets.

Healthy Portions

One of the major problems that also influences diabetic control and the weight epidemic in the US and the Western world is the quantity of food we eat during a meal. Abundance, especially in food, is a central part of celebration for any society. However, overeating at mealtime has become the norm rather than the exception. Even when eating good quality foods, if you eat too much your body will need to store the excess as fat.

We are almost all guilty of large portions, which are frequently followed with a second helping. The majority of restaurants today are focusing more on the *quantity* of food they serve rather than the *quality* of food to convince their customers to return. Chinese food, Mexican food, Italian food, and many other cultural restaurants are known for their large servings or family style approach. Eating at home is not necessarily better in this regard. Family style eating is very conducive to eating more than one serving of everything. This needs to change!

Following a heavy meal, there is a large shunting of blood to the gastrointestinal (GI) tract to help carry away all the calories we have just eaten. Most of us have felt the overwhelming feeling of sluggishness following such a meal. This is primarily related to the shifting of the blood supply to our gut. This is when most of us would rather take a nap than do the dishes or return to work.

When you eat the right amount and the right kind of food, you will be neither hungry nor stuffed, especially if you learn to eat your meals and snacks slowly allowing your brain to catch up to your stomach and tell your body that has had enough nourishment. You will feel satisfied and actually experience a surge of energy and focus for three to four hours following this meal. Eating smaller, more frequent meals when compared to eating one or two large meals daily has actually been shown to increase weight loss and diabetic control. This leads us to a discussion on how frequently we should be eating.

Meal Frequency

Dr. David Jenkins, et al., reported in the *New England Journal of Medicine (NEJM)* that those who nibble all day long (17 snacks throughout the day) versus those who ate two meals daily (they ate the same amount of calories for the entire day) had lower cholesterol and LDL cholesterol levels as well as increased HDL cholesterol levels. Insulin levels also declined and there was an overall improvement in all the cardiovascular risk factors. Other studies relate to the fact that when you only eat 1 or 2 meals daily, you actually gain more weight even if the amount of total calories you eat remains the same. Furthermore, clinical studies indicate that those individuals who skip breakfast actually gain more weight than those individuals who eat breakfast.

It is not practical with our busy schedules to eat 8 to 17 snacks daily, but you can accomplish the same benefits by eating three low-glycemic meals daily along with one or two low-glycemic snacks. It is important that you never become too hungry anytime during the day. This will almost always lead to overeating during the next meal. **Remember, food is one of the greatest drugs you ingest into your body.** Eating frequent, well-balanced meals and snacks is the key to feeling great throughout the day and improving insulin resistance and diabetic control.

MODEST EXERCISE PROGRAM

Have you ever stopped to consider the amazing strength and flexibility of the body as well as the feats of human strength throughout the history of mankind? It's mind-boggling to contemplate the hardships the body can endure! Consider the challenges faced by ancient nomadic people who crossed great expanses of land, or even the accomplishments of our immigrant forefathers and mothers in spite of: drought, rushing rivers, starvation, blizzards, freezing temperatures, wild predators, desert sandstorms, merciless seas, and rugged mountain tops. Through it all the body survives; miraculously the body overcomes and grows stronger still. Yet there is one adversity the human body cannot conquer—inactivity.

A study published last year in *The New England Journal of Medicine* indicated that *physical inactivity* might actually be more harmful to your health than other familiar risk factors, such as smoking, hypertension, and cardiovascular disease. The leading author of this study, Jonathan Myers, PhD, stated in the July 2003 issue of *Prevention* magazine, "Our study showed that a person's exercise capacity, measured by their ability to perform on a treadmill, was a more powerful predictor of mortality than all other risk factors. It also showed that, regardless of any other risk factors you have, if you're physically fit, you can cut your risk of premature death in half." In addition, those who were in excellent physical shape, no matter what their sport, did not have any evidence of insulin resistance or type 2 diabetes mellitus.

The one thing that flies in the face of our marvelous design is immobility. By design our bodies not only have the ability of great strength and stamina, they *require* physical challenge. We are designed to work and play hard. I once heard that 90 % of humanity for 90% of human history has spent 90% of their time hauling water and securing a roof over their heads. This puts life into perspective doesn't it? Our bodies were designed to withstand physical hardship.

On the other hand, we were not fashioned to endure great amounts of mental and emotional stress while leaving our bodies virtually motionless. With the rise of technology, we could easily seal our own fate. The human body cannot endure the life of immobility many of us know. We wake up, shower, walk to the car, drive to the parking garage at the office, take the elevator up, walk three doors down to the cubical, sit all day at a desk resolving stressful conflicts, eat a sandwich while working over lunch, get off an hour early to beat the traffic jam home, walk three doors down to the elevator, drive, walk into the living room, and watch television.

The very phrase "I need to exercise," begs the question, doesn't it? After all, we must eat, sleep, and move. How disappointing to discover that the term, "exercise," has taken on the same miserable fallacy as the word, "diet" in our American culture. Diet is not some torturous 21-day regime we embark on, nor is our need for exercise a 30-minute scheduled event. Eating delicious food and moving without pain are two of life's greatest pleasures. Not only are we born with the ability to choose what to eat and where we will go, our bodies can do so with strength, agility, speed and creativity. We are alive! This is what we do!

EXERCISE IMPROVES INSULIN SENSITIVITY

Now that you realize insulin resistance is the root problem for the overwhelming majority of individuals who have diabetes or who are struggling with their weight, we will continue our journey on learning how you can reverse this devastating problem. Physical activity (aka exercise) is one of the three pillars needed to accomplish this goal. You don't have to be a marathon runner; rather, consistent brisk walking is one of the central components of the Healthy for Life Program. Several studies have provided scientific data revealing how even modest exercise improves insulin resistance. It is important for us to review these studies so that you can learn to be more effective in choosing which exercise program or programs are appropriate for you.

Physical Training and Insulin Sensitivity

Well-trained athletes have one common characteristic—they all have low plasma insulin levels and are extremely sensitive to insulin. It does not seem to matter in which activity or sport these athletes are involved, rather being in excellent physical condition does have its definite health benefits.

Weight lifters and those primarily involved in anaerobic (weight resistant exercise) have somewhat improved glucose handling because of their increase in muscle mass. Since 80% to 90% of the blood glucose is normally taken up by the muscle cells, these athletes have more muscle to do so. In fact, in most studies these individuals have 35% greater muscle mass than the control population of sedentary individuals. It is important to remember that when we first develop insulin resistance, the muscle becomes resistant to insulin first, which then diverts the sugar to the fat cells of the abdomen where the sugar is turned into fat. Therefore, the more muscle we have to take up and utilize the sugar, the less will turn to fat.

Runners or athletes who are primarily involved in aerobic exercise, on the other hand, handle glucose even better than weight lifters because of their overall enhanced insulin sensitivity. Therefore, it is believed that aerobic exercise is actually more important in reversing insulin resistance than weight resistant exercises. However, there are many good reasons to have both aerobic and weight resistant activity in your exercise program.

The Power of Physical Activity

Studies have looked at individuals who were previously sedentary and totally out of shape and then observed them when they began to exercise. These clinical studies reveal that insulin sensitivity improves directly in proportion to the improvement in physical fitness. This is important to note because a majority of people interested in controlling their diabetes or weight loss have not been in good physical condition for quite some time. You will find that when developing these new lifestyle habits, the body has a remarkable ability to change; **most of the medical problems and weight gain brought on by poor eating habits and a sedentary lifestyle can be reversed.** It is important to know that even though intensive activity can significantly enhance insulin sensitivity, modest, long-term physical activity (like walking) is also very effective in reversing insulin resistance.

No matter what your age or physical condition, medical evidence strongly supports the fact that modest physical training can improve one's sensitivity to insulin. This improvement is directly related to aerobic exercise, not as a result of weight loss as many in the medical community believe. This means that reversing insulin resistance allows the body to "tip back" into a normal metabolic state so that it can utilize the calories you consume normally. Therefore, when you see a chart that shows how many calories you have expended doing a certain activity, don't get discouraged. It is not the concept of calories in must equal calories out that is critical for weight loss. It is improving and reversing insulin resistance so that the body can release fat that is critical. Then your body will begin to release the fat that it has been holding onto so tightly. You are going to gain much more in terms of health benefits and weight loss than the mere calories you use up doing a particular activity. In other words, the gains you receive from merely having a modest, consistent exercise program are dramatic compared to the amount of exercise you really do. This is even truer with people who have diabetes or who are becoming diabetic. A simple, consistent exercise program is essential if you have any desire to improve or protect your health.

Modest Exercise for Individuals who are Overweight

The evidence in clinical trials showing insulin resistance in those who are obese is primarily due to the lack of sensitivity to insulin in the *muscle tissue.* After the muscle tissue is stimulated through exercise, overweight individuals become significantly more responsive to insulin in their muscle and their bodies are able to again take up the glucose from the blood stream and utilize it in their muscles rather than have it diverted to the adipose or fat tissue.

Dr. A. S. Leon et al. studied the effect of modest exercise (brisk walking for 15 to 90 minutes five times weekly) in previously sedentary, overweight individuals. When the study group was again evaluated after 16 weeks into the program, *all* were found to have a significant increase (nearly 50%) in sensitivity to their own insulin. An average fat loss of 13 pounds was reported as a result of the clinical trial.

How Exercise Effects Insulin Sensitivity

Exercise has several positive effects on insulin sensitivity, which helps restore the normal response to insulin.

1. The capillary bed (the small blood vessels) in the muscle actually dilates and creates significantly more blood flow to the muscle. As you will recall, one of the first problems leading to insulin resistance is the vasoconstriction (narrowing of the arteries) of this capillary bed in the muscle, which decreases the blood flow to the muscle and creates a physical barrier for insulin to pass through to the surrounding tissue and cells.

2. Exercise is the key in promoting this circulation to the muscle tissue. This allows much more insulin to actually get to the muscle cell. Transport of glucose into the muscle cell is greatly increased. This is due to an enhancement of the post-receptor site transport of glucose.

3. Physical training has been found to increase muscle tissue sensitivity to insulin in proportion to the improvement of physical fitness.

Developing a Consistent,
Effective Personal Exercise Program

There have been several truths that I have learned over my thirty years of clinical practice, especially when it comes to directing and encouraging my patients to make some healthy lifestyle changes. First, the approach to an exercise program must be practical and achievable. Second, he or she must understand the importance of developing a consistent and effective exercise program, which is much easier than most people realize. This is especially true when it comes to my diabetic patients. Obviously, lack of exercise is one of the major reasons they have become diabetic in the first place. Third, they need to be encouraged to take the steps that are necessary to successfully accomplish their goal of improved health and permanent fat loss.

Approach

In order for aerobic exercise to have any beneficial effect on insulin resistance and in turn, fat loss, an individual needs to build up to brisk exercise greater than 30 minutes, five times weekly. I say "five times weekly" because your body also needs rest and time to rejuvenate itself, especially if you've had little activity in months past. Improving strength, stamina, and endurance requires that your muscles and body receive quality rest during your week.

Consistent and Effective

It is critical; however, to exercise a minimum of at least three days per week or little will be accomplished. Habitual aerobic exercise is absolutely necessary if you desire to have any hope of significantly decreasing your risk of diabetes, controlling your diabetes, or achieving permanent fat loss. Think of it this way: the doctor has prescribed that you get out of your mundane routine and have some fun!

You must enjoy the exercise program as much as is humanly possible and exercise in an atmosphere where you are totally comfortable. This may not be a gym, a health club, or anywhere in public. Many people are self-conscious about their bodies and do not want to go to an environment they perceive as competitive and uncomfortable. On the other hand, there are a number of people who need to join a health club or YMCA because they enjoy working out with other people or need the encouragement and support of a group exercise program. The important thing is that you choose an exercise program that is comfortable for you and one that you will enjoy.

Successfully Accomplish Your Goals

I am not speaking as a fitness guru. I am a physician concerned about safe exercise for complete body health. For the majority of my patients, I recommend they begin with a simple walking program because it is generally easier, low-impact, and does not require spending any extra money on equipment or health club dues. Some patients choose to ride their bike, jog, swim, play tennis or racquetball, or join an aerobic exercise group at their local health club.

A blend of activities is even better. Choose a couple or several different aerobic exercise activities to work into your exercise program. For instance, you may play tennis twice a week and walk while playing golf three times a week. I personally like a blend of weight resistance with a more aggressive aerobic workout either done together or on different days of the week. Needless to say, you will not have the success you desire without developing a consistent, but modest, exercise program.

If you are over 40 and have not been very active for several years, I strongly recommend that you consult your physician before you begin an exercise program. If you are dealing with an old or new injury, you may want to be referred to a physical therapist or chiropractor for guidance into the best exercise program that would not aggravate that injury.

Starting slow and building up to the recommended level of exercise is also critical. Most of you have been out of shape for years. Remember, it is the long-term goal of getting back into shape that is critical. Even if you are only able to walk 5 to 10 minutes at a slow pace, that is just fine. Your body will adjust and respond to even this level of activity. It just a matter of a short period of time of a month or two you will be able to slowly build up to the recommended level. Once you are able to walk at a comfortable pace for 30 minutes five days a week, then you can try to increase your pace to what I refer to as brisk walking. You can take these same principles and apply them to any exercise program you may have chosen to pursue. The last thing you want to do is to hurt yourself and not be able to exercise for weeks at a time.

CELLULAR NUTRITION

My book, *What Your Doctor Doesn't Know about Nutritional Medicine* (Thomas Nelson, 2002) details the problem of oxidative stress and the solution, which is cellular nutrition. Here I am only able to give brief highlights in regards to diabetics and the prevention of diabetes. If you would like more complete information, I encourage you to obtain a copy of this book so you can learn more about the astounding health benefits offered by nutritional supplementation. However, cellular nutrition is a critical aspect of the Healthy for Life Program and is essential in improving insulin sensitivity.

Oxidative Stress

The medical literature is beginning to address how the root or underlying cause of over 70 chronic degenerative diseases like heart disease, stroke, cancer, diabetes, arthritis, Alzheimer dementia and even insulin resistance is oxidative stress. Initially, oxidative stress attacks the capillary bed within the muscle, which then creates inflammation and vasoconstriction (narrowing of the arteries) making it more difficult for insulin to pass from the blood stream to the cell where it is able to perform its job.

What is oxidative stress? As the body utilizes oxygen needed to sustain life itself, occasionally a charged oxygen molecule is produced called a free radical. This oxygen molecule has at least one unpaired electron in its outer orbit, which gives it an electrical charge. A highly reactive oxygen molecule created by the electrical charge moves rapidly in its quest to find an additional electron from any source nearby. If this free radical is not neutralized by an antioxidant (which has the ability to give this free radical an additional electron and render it harmless), it can go on to create even more volatile free radicals. As free radicals increase, damage is done to the cell wall, vessel wall, proteins, fats and even the DNA nucleus of the cell.

We are not defenseless against this attack by these free radicals. However, we must have enough antioxidants available to handle the number of free radicals produced. If not, oxidative stress occurs and the body is vulnerable to degeneration similar to rust on a car. The body produces some antioxidants and we are able to get additional antioxidants from our foods—primarily from fruits and vegetables. When enough antioxidants are "on board," to handle the number of free radicals you are producing the body is protected. It all becomes a matter of balance.

The number of free radicals produced is never constant; there are many situations and conditions that increase the number of free radicals you produce. Excessive emotional stress or exercise, pollutants in our air, food and water, cigarette smoke, medications, sunlight, and radiation all cause our bodies to produce excessive amounts of free radicals. Because of our stressful lifestyles, polluted environment, and poor diet the medical literature strongly supports the need to supplement our diet with a wide variety of different antioxidants and their supporting minerals and vitamin B cofactors.

Our Food: Ally or Enemy?

Undoubtedly, what we eat has a profound and lasting influence on our health. As you are learning, food becomes either our greatest ally or our greatest enemy. The decision is ours. As you may recall, medical researchers are finding the period of time that occurs shortly after the meal—called the *postprandial state*—to be absolutely the most critical to the body's well-being, especially for the diabetic. In previous sections I have touched upon the events that follow a high-glycemic meal. Here I will briefly set the stage again so you can see how effective nutritional supplements are in reversing oxidative stress caused by our eating habits.

ANTIOXIDANT SUPPLEMENTS—THE ANSWER

It is true that combining good low-glycemic carbohydrates, with good fat, and good protein in each meal is one of the pillars of success. It is important to realize that, in addition, consuming antioxidant supplements (another pillar) with each meal not only protects your arteries but is essential for lasting, vibrant health (and of course diabetic control and fat loss). There have now been several studies, which reveal convincing data that supplemental vitamin C and vitamin E are able to reverse endothelial dysfunction caused by the elevated blood sugars in diabetic patients and patients with coronary artery disease!

Vitamin C

Vitamin C is the best antioxidant located within the plasma or blood. It also has the ability to easily neutralize the superoxide free radical that is created by hyperglycemia (elevated blood sugars) and elevated triglycerides. When vitamin C is given in supplementation to diabetic patients who already have significant endothelial dysfunction they showed marked improvement.

Vitamin C also has the ability to regenerate vitamin E. Dr. Antonio Ceriello makes special note of the fact that antioxidants work together in the body and it is hard to separate them out and try to study them individually. He states, "These antioxidants act synergistically in vivo (in the body), so as to provide the organism with a greater protection against radical damage than any single antioxidant can provide by itself." Therefore, it becomes important to look at all these studies as showing just a glimpse of the total picture that is actually occurring inside the body. This is one of the main reasons that I promote the concept of cellular nutrition.

Vitamin E

Vitamin E is the most potent antioxidant within the cell membrane. In fact, several studies have shown that vitamin E is able to incorporate itself into the wall of LDL cholesterol and help prevent it from becoming modified or oxidized. Dr. Paolisso, et al. also reported that optimal levels of vitamin E not only helped reduce the oxidative stress created by hyperglycemia and elevated triglycerides in the blood stream but it also improved insulin function. Vitamin E helps glucose transport as well as improves the pancreatic beta cell response to glucose and its subsequent production of insulin.

Chromium Supplementation

Chromium levels are not only critical for the proper functioning of insulin but also fat and glucose metabolism in the body. Almost all of our diabetic patients are very low in chromium and several studies have considered the benefits of giving diabetic patients chromium in supplementation. In fact, chromium is now routinely added to intravenous nutrition solutions used for very ill diabetic patients because of the results of these studies. Depending on the degree of insulin resistance or diabetes, individuals with insulin resistance tend to lose their ability to convert chromium into a usable form. This problem along with relative chromium deficiency appears to get worse in conjunction with the severity of insulin insensitivity or diabetes mellitus. There is also strong evidence that the intake of high-glycemic carbohydrates increases chromium loss.

Supplemental chromium leads to an increased binding of insulin to the receptor sites of the cell. There is also evidence that chromium allows insulin to be more active and effective in doing its job. Chromium has also been shown to make the pancreatic beta cells more sensitive for the effective release of insulin. Dr. Anderson concludes that the overall effect of supplemental chromium is to increase insulin sensitivity, which leads to helping reverse the metabolic syndrome.

Magnesium Supplementation

Magnesium plays a very important role in glucose metabolism within the body because just like chromium it affects both insulin secretion and action. It has been demonstrated in many studies that as people age, their magnesium levels decrease. This phenomenon is seen in both the non-diabetic and diabetic patients who also suffer from increasing insulin resistance. Dr.

Paolisso and his group studied how supplemental magnesium improved insulin secretion and enhanced insulin action. They also found evidence that daily magnesium supplements improved the cell wall membrane and increased intracellular potassium levels. Daily magnesium supplementation again improved insulin resistance and all of its health consequences.

Other Micronutrients

Several other micronutrients have been studied in patients with insulin resistance and diabetes mellitus as well. Dr. Thompson and Dr. Godin reviewed the medical literature and found strong evidence that supplementing their patients' diet with zinc, manganese, glutathione, selenium, and vanadium improved insulin sensitivity. They point out that studies involving vanadium have drawn increasing interest over the past few years because of its ability to improve insulin sensitivity when given at optimal levels.

Cellular Nutrition

The last section was highly technical, but I wanted you to have the evidence that demands a verdict—should you be taking nutritional supplements if your goal is either to prevent or reverse diabetes? Cellular nutrition enhances our antioxidant defense system, our immune system, and our body's repair system. This provides the best overall chance of preventing oxidative stress and protecting our health as we are improving insulin resistance. Nowhere is cellular nutrition more important than in helping prevent or reversing insulin resistance and diabetes.

Dr. Das wrote an editorial in *Nutrition* wherein he points out a common thread between obesity, the metabolic syndrome, and inflammation. He believes that the metabolic syndrome is due to a low-grade systemic inflammation which leads to insulin resistance and the harmful metabolic changes and related obesity. There is strong clinical evidence that individuals with the metabolic syndrome, (including central obesity), have elevated blood levels of C-reactive protein (CRP), tumor necrosis factor-alpha (TNA-alpha) and interluekin-6 (IL-6)—all markers of inflammation in the body. I couldn't agree more. Oxidative stress is the underlying cause of this inflammation.

The best way to accomplish this goal is to consume what I refer to as cellular nutrition. Cellular nutrition is defined as consuming all of these micronutrients in supplementation at these optimal levels or levels that have been shown to provide a health benefit in our medical literature. By providing these optimal levels of supplementation, you not only are able to replenish any deficiency but you are also able to bring all the necessary nutrients up to their optimal levels. These nutrients work together against a variety of different free radicals in different parts of the body. By simply consuming a high-quality, complete and balanced nutritional supplement, you can easily accomplish the third pillar of a healthy lifestyle—nutritional supplementation. So what should you consider in choosing a nutritional supplement that will provide all of these health benefits?

PHARMACEUTICAL-GRADE GOOD MANUFACTURING PRACTICES (GMP)

When you are considering which nutritional supplements to take, there are a few important criteria you need to consider before choosing a particular brand of supplement in order to get the quality you need.

The nutritional supplement industry is basically an unregulated industry. The FDA considers nutritional supplements in the same category as a food. This means there is no guarantee that what is on the label is actually in the tablet. You need to select a company that manufactures their products as if they were a drug and not a food. The companies that accomplish this goal follow what is known as pharmaceutical-grade Good Manufacturing Practices (GMP). This means they purchase pharmaceutical grade raw products and then produce them with the same quality control that a pharmaceutical company does. Nutritional companies are not required to do this, but a few of the companies are now strictly following these guidelines so they can offer you the assurance that what they have listed on the label is in fact, what is in the tablet.

US Pharmacopoeia (USP)

Your tablets must readily dissolve or it really doesn't matter what is in them. When nutritional companies follow these USP guidelines, it gives you the assurance that at least your tablet is dissolving. Still many nutritional companies do not follow USP guidelines. The government is definitely getting more serious about trying to raise the bar on the quality of nutritional supplements in this country and the FDA is now looking into setting higher standards for the production of nutritional supplements. However, this will take several more years to implement.

Complete and Balanced

Your nutritional supplements need to be complete and balanced. What I mean by this is that they provide the optimal (not RDA levels) levels of several different antioxidants and their supporting B-cofactors (vitamin B1, B2, B5, B6, B12, and folic acid) along with the so-called antioxidant minerals (selenium, magnesium, zinc, copper, manganese, chromium, and vanadium). When you begin to realize the significant health benefits you can receive from nutritional supplementation, you also begin to see the importance of a complete and balanced supplement that creates synergy. When all these nutrients are provided at these optimal or advanced levels, one plus one is not two, but instead, ten or twenty.

Synergy

Studies in the medical literature will usually single out one or two nutrients at a time. This is the common research method and is necessary for testing the effects of drugs. Nutritional supplements, on the other hand, are not in the same category and must be considered otherwise. For example, Vitamins E or C are not drugs but rather nutrients we should be getting from our foods. However, because of supplementation we are now able to get these nutrients at optimal levels you could never obtain from your food.

When testing them, we must consider them together. Vitamin E is the best antioxidant within the cell membrane while vitamin C is the most efficient antioxidant within the plasma or blood. Glutathione is the leading intracellular antioxidant. Alpha lipoic acid is a great antioxidant within the plasma and the cell membrane; however, it also regenerates vitamin E and intracellular glutathione so they can be used over and over again. Vitamin C also regenerates vitamin E. In addition, all of these antioxidants need optimal levels of B-cofactors and antioxidant minerals in order to do their job efficiently. When you put all of this together, this is called synergy and this is what makes cellular nutrition so effective.

It is amazing to me how many studies show that you can receive a health benefit from simply taking one of these nutrients in supplementation. The overwhelming majority of these studies involving supplements show a definite health benefit. However, occasionally a study that looks at just supplementing one of these antioxidant nutrients has shown a negative result. This is due to the fact that when you supplement just one nutrient by itself at these optimal levels it can become a pro-oxidant, which means it can actually cause oxidative stress. By using the concept of cellular nutrition and providing all of these nutrients to the cell at these optimal levels, you not only enhance your body's natural immune, antioxidant, and repair system but you also are able to prevent any pro-oxidant affect produced by a single nutrient.

WHAT SUPPLEMENTS DO I RECOMMEND TO MY PATIENTS?

If you are serious about preventing diabetes or even reversing diabetes, I warn you to not sell yourself to the lowest bidder. You cannot possibly get everything you need by taking a multiple vitamin. Multiple vitamins are based on Recommended Daily Allowance (RDA) levels of supplementation. RDA's were developed in the late 1930's and 1940's as the minimal requirement needed to avoid acute deficiency diseases like pellagra, scurvy, or rickets. This standard has absolutely nothing to do with chronic degenerative diseases or insulin resistance. Please take time to look at Table 3.

There are companies that are putting almost all of these nutrients into one or two tablets that need to be taken 3 times daily. I encourage my patients to take an antioxidant tablet and mineral tablet with each meal. They need to contain as close to the amount of supplementation I recommend in Table 3. For my diabetic patients, I also encourage them to be taking 90mg of grape-seed extract twice daily along with at least two filtered fish oil capsules. Additional calcium and magnesium is also encouraged.

Table 3
Basic Nutritional Supplement Recommendations

ANTIOXIDANTS	The more and varied your antioxidants, the better.
VITAMIN A	I do not recommend the use of straight vitamin A because of its potential toxicity. I recommend supplementing with a mixture of mixed carotenoids. Carotenoids become vitamin A in the body as the body has need and they have no toxicity problems.
CAROTENOIDS	It is important to have a nice mixture of carotenoids and not just to take beta-carotene. • Beta-carotene — 10,000 to 15,000 IU • Lycopene — 1 to 3 mg • Lutein/Zeaxanthin — 1 to 6 mg • Alpha carotene — 500 mcg to 800 mcg
VITAMIN C	It is important to get a mixture of vitamin C, especially the calcium, potassium, zinc, and magnesium ascorbates, which are much more potent in handling oxidative stress. • 1000 to 2000 mg
VITAMIN E	It is important to be getting a mixture of vitamin Es. This should always be natural vitamin, and a mixture of natural vitamin is better: d-alpha tocopherol, d-gamma tocopherol, and mixed tocotrienol. • 400 to 800 IU
BIOFLAVANOID COMPLEX OF ANTIXODANTS	Bioflavanoids offer you a great variety of potent antioxidants. Having a variety of bioflavanoids is a great asset to your supplements. The amounts may vary but should include the majority of the following: • Rutin • Cruciferous • Quercitin • Bilberry • Broccoli • Grape-Seed Extract • Green Tea • Bromelain
ALPHA-LIPOIC ACID	• 15 to 30 mg
COQ10	• 20 to 30 mg
GLUTATHIONE	• 10 to 20 mg • Precursor: N-acetyl-L-cystein 50 to 75 mg
B VITAMINS (COFACTORS)	• Folic Acid — 800mcg • Vitamin B1 (Thiamin) — 20 to 30 mg • Vitamin B2 (Riboflavin) — 25 to 50 mg • Vitamin B3 (Niacin) — 30 to 75 mg • Vitamin B5 (Pantothenic Acid) — 80 to 200 mg • Vitamin B6 (Pyridoxine) — 25 to 50 mg • Vitamin B12 (Cobalamin) — 100mcg to 250 mcg • Biotin — 300mcg to 1,000 mcg

Table 3
Basic Nutritional Supplement Recommendations

OTHER IMPORTANT VITAMINS	• Vitamin D3 (Cholecalciferol) • Vitamin K 50 to 100mcg	450 IU to 800 IU
MINERAL COMPLEX	• Calcium	800 to 1,500 mg (depending on your dietary intake of calcium)
	• Magnesium	500 mg to 800 mg
	• Zinc	20 to 30 mg
	• Selenium	200 mcg is ideal
	• Chromium	200 mcg to 300 mcg
	• Copper1 to 3 mg	
	• Manganese	3 to 6 mg
	• Vanadium	30 to 100 mcg
	• Iodine 100 mcg to 200 mcg	
	• Molybdenum	50 mcg to 100 mcg
	• Mixture of Trace Minerals	
ADDITIONAL NUTRIENTS FOR BONE HEALTH	• Silicon 3 mg • Boron 2 to 3 mg	
OTHER IMPORTANT AND ESSENTIAL NUTRIENTS Improved Homocysteine levels and improved brain function	• Choline • Trimethylglycine • Inositol 150 mg to 250 mg	100 to 200 mg 200 to 500 mg
SUPPLEMENTING YOUR DIET		
ESSENTIAL FATS:	• Cold-Pressed Flaxseed oil • Fish Oil Capsules	
FIBER SUPPLEMENT	• Blend of soluble and insoluble fiber	10 to 30 mg depending on your dietary comsumption fiber (ideal is 35 to 50 grams of total fiber daily)

**There are some nutritional companies who are putting together these essential nutrients into one or two different tablets, which need to be taken 2 to 3 times daily in order to achieve this level of supplementation. Look for a high-quality product that comes as close as possible to these recommendations. If the manufacturer follows pharmaceutical GMP and USP guidelines, you will be giving yourself the absolute best protection against oxidative stress.

The essential fats and fiber will give you the added nutrients that are usually missing in the Western diet.

HEALTHY FOR LIFE PROGRAM LOCATED AT www.ReleasingFat.com

Now that more and more people are beginning to become proactive with their health they want to know what they can do that will truly be clinically effective. In this sea of information, people become more and more confused the more they read. If you are going to spend all this time, money, and effort on trying to improve your lifestyle, wouldn't you want it to be clinically effective? Changing lifestyle behavior is not an easy task. In fact, I have dedicated the last 12 years of my medical practice learning what it takes to help people accomplish their goal of establishing these new, healthier lifestyles that give them the best possible chance of preventing diabetes or even possibly reversing diabetes. This is why the Healthy for Life Program was developed. It is a 15-month program that takes you by the hand and educates you, motivates you, and holds you accountable to these new, healthier lifestyles that have been shown to be clinically effective. You can choose either the "Coached" program, where you are assigned your own personal lifestyle coach, or the more affordable "Self-Directed" program. In both programs, you will receive daily emails from me along with weekly trainings for the first 12 weeks of the program and weekly emails and monthly advanced trainings during the last 12 months. You can either read these trainings or view a "flash audio presentation."

You will have your own personal lifestyle journal where you will record exactly what you are eating, how you are taking your nutritionals, and how you are exercising. Simply writing down what you are actually doing in regards to your lifestyle allows these subconscious lifestyle habits to become conscious. This allows you to deal with them honestly. What you will learn very quickly is that you do not have to be perfect to have success in this program; however, you must be honest with yourself. Over the 15 months of the program, these new healthier lifestyles will eventually become unconscious again; however, this time they will be good lifestyle habits. This journal is automatically graded; however, it is also reviewed periodically by your coach in the "Coached" program.

You must remember this is not a diet, but instead, is the beginning of establishing these new healthier lifestyles. However, there is one word of caution for the diabetic patient. You must follow your blood sugars carefully. I would recommend checking your blood sugars at least 4 times daily with your glucometer.

Participants are encouraged to begin with Phase 1 of the Healthy for Life program. In Phase 1 you replace two meals and one snack daily with meal and snack replacements that are known to be low-glycemic. There are companies that are now producing high-quality meal and snack replacements that are definitely low-glycemic. You also have one regular low-glycemic snack and one regular low-glycemic meal. You need to avoid all breads, flour, rice, pasta, cereals, sugar, and potatoes during Phase 1 of the program. These are the most likely foods that will spike your blood sugar and quickly set off this carbohydrate addiction again. Again, if you are hungry, you simply eat another low-glycemic meal or snack. You also need to begin a modest, consistent exercise program along with providing the body with the cellular nutrition I recommend.

Once you are well along in reaching your personal health and weight goals, you would move on to Phase 2. In Phase 2 of the Healthy for Life Program you have two regular low-glycemic meals and one regular low-glycemic snack along with one low-glycemic meal and one low-glycemic snack replacement. You will also begin adding back those healthy, whole grain breads and cereals along with the lower-glycemic rice and potatoes into your diet.

You would also slowly increase the intensity of your workouts along with continuing your nutritional supplements, which allows you the best opportunity to **RESET Your Life** and reverse any insulin resistance. It allows the individual to "tip back" into their normal metabolic state.

I have learned over 30 years of clinical practice and through countless studies reported in our medical literature, that diets simply do not work. In fact, they fail 98% of the time. This is because they are a short-term solution for a long-term problem. They are also generally not balanced diets or healthy diets. But the main reason they do not work is because they don't correct the underlying problem, which is insulin resistance. Remember, the Healthy for Life Program is not a diet. These are healthy lifestyles you must continue the rest of your life, which will then provide a side effect of permanent weight loss. However, I have found that you must continue this program for at least 15 months to firmly establish these new, healthier lifestyles. Remember, these are healthy lifestyles that you want to be doing for the rest of your life.

I would encourage each and every one of you to visit my web site located at **www.releasingfat.com** and check out this amazing Internet site. Take a look at the overview of the program and the web site tour to learn more about how this site is able to help you achieve these new healthier lifestyles. Also take advantage of the FREE "Automated Health Risk Assessment" that I have developed. You can find out if you already have any evidence of insulin resistance. Knowing this information is great; however, it is very difficult to change lifestyles that you have established over a lifetime. This is why it is critical to consider becoming a member of this web page and allowing us to take you by the hand and educate you, motivate you, and hold you accountable to these new, healthier lifestyles.

This program has been shown to be clinically effective in two separate clinical trials. The last study was done under the supervision and guidelines of the Western International Review Board and FDA. Twenty-five participants who showed evidence of early insulin resistance were involved in this twelve-week study. They participated in Phase 1 and 2 of the Healthy for Life Program and were followed at **www.releasingfat.com.** Within twelve weeks they had an average weight loss of 13 pounds, they decreased their body mass index (BMI) by 2.2 points, and they lost an average of 2¹/₂ inches off their waist measurements. Their systolic blood pressure (the high number) dropped an average 10 points and their diastolic pressure (the low number) dropped an average of 6 points. Their total cholesterol dropped an average of 17%, the LDL cholesterol dropped an average of 19%, and their triglyceride levels dropped an average of 23%. This was all the result of improved insulin sensitivity, which improved over 12%. As you would expect, their insulin levels dropped an amazing 40% during the 12 weeks of the study.

Physicians, chiropractors, osteopaths, health clubs, and naturopaths across the country are now incorporating the Healthy for Life Program into their practices and health clubs. It offers their patients and clients an opportunity to develop these healthy lifestyles that have been shown to be clinically effective. If you have a desire to prevent ever becoming diabetic or improving your diabetes, if you are already diabetic, then you want to strongly consider applying this cutting-edge scientific information to your life. The easiest way to accomplish this goal is to become a participant of the Healthy for Life Program today. Check it out at **www.releasingfat.com** and begin taking back control of your health.

REFERENCES

Allred, J.B. "Too Much of a Good Thing? An Overemphasis on Eating Low-Fat Foods May be Contributing to the Alarming Increase in Overweight Among US Adults." *Journal of the American Diet Association* 95. (1995): 417-418.

American Diabetes Association. "Type 2 Diabetes in Children and Adolescents." *Diabetes Care 22.* (2000): 381-389.

Bantle, J.P., et al. "Postprndial Glucose and Insulin Responses to Meals Containing Different Carbohydrates in Normal and Diabetic Subjects." *New England Journal of Medicine* 309. (1983): 7-12.

Bjorntorp, P., et al. "The Glucose Uptake of Human Adipose Tissue in Obesity." *European Journal of Clinical Investigation* 1. (1971): 480-485.

Bjorntorp, P., et al. "The Effect of Physical Training on Insulin Production in Obesity." *Metabolism* 19. (1970): 631-638.

Blanco, I., and S.B. Roberts. "High Glycemic Index Foods, Over-Eating, and Obesity." *Pediatrics* 103. (1999): E261-E266.

Block G. Dietary guidelines and the results of food surveys. *American Journal of Clinical Nutrition* 53 (1991): 3565-75

Brand, J.C., et al. "The Glycemic Index is Easy and Works in Practice." *Diabetes Care* 20. (1997): 1628-1629.

Ceriello, A., et al. "Meal Induced Oxidative Stress and Low-Density Lipoprotein Oxidation in Diabetes: The Possible Role of Hyperglycemia." *Metabolism* 48. (1999): 1503-1508.

Ceriello, A., and M. Pirisi. "Is Oxidative Stress the Missing Link Between Insulin Resistance and Atherosclerosis?" (letter). *Diabetologia* 38. (1995): 1484-1485.

Cooper, K, "Antioxidant Revolution", 94-10134 CIP, Thomas Nelson Publishing 1994.

Das, U. "Obesity, Metabolic Syndrome X, and Inflammation." *Nutrition* 18. (2001): 430-432.

Davies, Calvin. "Oxidative stress: The paradox of aerobic life." Biochem Soc Symp 61 (1995): 1-31

Davies K, "Oxidative Stress, Antioxidant Defenses, and Damage Removal, Repair and Replacement Systems." Life, 50:279-289 2000.

Evans, D.J., et al. "Relationship Between Skeletal Muscle Insulin Resistance, Insulin-Mediated Glucose Disposal, and Insulin Binding: Effects of Obesity and Body Fat Topography." *Journal of Clinical Investigation* 74. (1984): 1515-1525.

Flegal, K.M., et al. "Overweight and Obesity in the US: Prevalence and Trends, 1960-1994." *International Journal of Obesity* 22. (1998): 39-47.

Fontaine, K.R., et al. "Years of Life Lost Due to Obesity." *JAMA* 289. (2003): 187-193.

Ford, E.S., et al. "Prevalence of the Metabolic Syndrome Among US Adults." *JAMA* 287 (2002): 356-359.

Foster-Powell, K., and J.B. Miller. "International Tables of Glycemic Index." *American Journal of Clinical Nutrition* 62. (1995): 871S-890S.

Foster-Powell, K., Brand-Miller, J.C, and Holt, S.H.A. "International Table of Glycemic Index and Glycemic Load Values: 2002." *American Journal of Clinical Nutrition* 76, (2002): 5-56.

Helmrich, S.P., et al. "Physical Activity and Reduced Occurrence of Non-Insulin Dependent Diabetes Mellitus." *New England Journal of Medicine* 325. (1991): 147-152.

Holloszy, J.O., et.al. "Effects of Exercise on Glucose Tolerance and Insulin Resistance." *Acta Medica Scandinavica* 711. (1996): 55-65.

Holt, S., et al "Relationship of Satiety to Postprandial Glycaemic, Insulin and Cholecystokinin Responses." *Appetite* 18. (1992): 129-141.

Hu, FB, et al. "Television Watching and Other Sedentary Behaviors in Relation to Risk of Obesity and Type 2 Diabetes Mellitus in Women." *JAMA* 289, (2003): 1785-1791.

Koivisto, V., and R.A. DeFronzo. "Physical Training and Insulin Sensitivity." *Diabetes Metabolism Reviews* 1. (1986): 445-481.

Jenkins, D., et al. "Glycemic Index of Foods: A Physiological Basis for Carbohydrate Exchange." *American Journal of Clinical Nutrition* 34. (1981): 362-366.

Jenkins, D., et al. "Nibbling Versus, Gorging: Metabolic Advantages of Increased Meal Frequency." *New England Journal of Medicine* 321. (1989): 929-934.

Lawrence, M., et al. "Oral Glucose Loading Acutely Attenuates Endothelium-Dependent Vasodilation in Healthy Adults Without Diabetes: An Effect Prevented by Vitamins C and E. *Journal of the American College of Cardiology* 36. (2000): 2185-2191.

Leathwood, P., Pollet, P. "Effects of Slow Release Carbohydrates in the Form of Bean Flakes on the Evolution of Hunger and Satiety in Man." *Appetite* 10. (1988): 1-11.

Leon, A.S., et al. "Effects of Vigorous Walking Program on Body Composition, and Carbohydrate and Lipid Metabolism of Obese Young Men." *Journal of Clinical Nutrition* 33 (1979):1776-1787.

Ludwig, D.S., et al. "High Glycemic Index Foods, Overeating, and Obesity." *Pediatrics* 103. (1999): e26.

Ludwig, D.S. "The Glycemic Index: Physiological Mechanisms Relating to Obesity, Diabetes, and Cardiovascular Disease." *JAMA* 287. (2002): 2412-2423.

Martin-Moreno, J., et al. "Dietary Fat, Olive Oil Intake and Breast Cancer Risk." *International Journal of Cancer* 58. (1994): 774-780.

Mayer-Davis, E.J., et al. "Intensity and Amount of Physical Activity in Relation to Insulin Sensitivity." *JAMA* 279. (1998): 669-674

Moller P., H. Wallin, and L. Knudsen. "Oxidative stress associated with exercise, psychological stress, and life-style factors." Chemico-Biological Interactions 102 (1996): 17-36.

Nuttall, F.Q., et al. "Effect of Protein Ingestion on the Glucose and Insulin Response to a Standardized Oral Glucose Load." *Diabetes Care* 7. (1984): 465-70.

Pinkey, J.A., et al. "Endothelial Cell Dysfunction: Cause of the Insulin Resistance Syndrome." *Diabetes* 46. (1997): S9-S13.

Reaven, G.M. "Syndrome X: 6 Years Later." *Journal of Internal Medicine Suppl* 736. (1994): 13-22.

Ross, R., "Atherosclerosis-an Inflammatory Disease." *New England Journal of Medicine* 340, (1999): 115-123.

Rossetti, L., et al. "Glucose Toxicity." *Diabetes Care* 13. (1990): 610-630.

Schlosser, Eric. *Fast Food Nation,* Mifflin Company, (2002).

Subar, A.F., et al. "Dietary Sources of Nutrients Among US Children, 1989-1991." *Pediatrics* 102. (1998): 913-923.

Torjesen, P.A., et al. "Lifestyle Changes May Reverse Development of the Insulin Resistance Syndrome." *Diabetes Care* 30. (1997): 26-31.

Troiano, R.P., et al. "Overweight Prevalence and Trends for Children and Adolescents: The National Health and Nutrition Examination Surveys, 1963-1991." *Arch Pediatric. Adolesc. Med.* 149. (1995): 1085-1091.

Visioli, F., and C. Galli. "Olive Oil Phenols and Their Potential Effects on Human Health." *Journal of Agnc. Food Chem.* 46. (1998): 42922-4296.

Weil, Andrew, *Eating Well for Optimal Health.* Alfred A. Knopf (2000)

Willett, W., et al. "Mediterranean Diet Pyramid: A Cultural Model for Healthy Eating." *American Journal of Clinical Nutrition* 61. (1995): 1402S-1406S.

Wolever, T., et al. "The Glycemic Index: Methodology and Clinical Implications." *American Journal of Clinical Nutrition* 54. (1991): 846-854.

Strand, Ray. *What Your Doctor Doesn't Know About Nutritional Medicine May Be Killing You.* Thomas Nelson Publishers. (2002).

Thompson, K.H., and D.V. Godlin. "Micronutrients and Antioxidants in the Progression of Diabetes." *Nutrition Research* 15. (1995): 1377-1410.

Yamanouchi, K.T., et al. "Daily Walking Combined with Diet Therapy is Useful Means for Obese NIDDM Patients Not Only to Reduce Body Weight But Also to Improve Insulin Sensitivity." *Diabetes Care* 18. (1995): 775-778.

Young IS, "Antioxidants in health and disease." J Clin Pathol 2001 Mar; 54(3):176-86.

ABOUT THE AUTHOR

Ray D. Strand, M. D., graduated from the University of Colorado Medical School and finished his post-graduate training at Mercy Hospital in San Diego, California. He has been involved in an active private family practice for the past thirty years, and has focused his practice on nutritional medicine over the past ten years while lecturing internationally on the subject. He is also the author of several best-selling books that includes *What Your Doctor Doesn't Know About Nutritional Medicine, Death by Prescription, Living By Design,* and *Releasing Fat.* He has also lectured across the United States, Canada, Australia, and New Zealand on preventive and nutritional medicine. Dr. Strand lives on a horse ranch in South Dakota with his lovely wife, Elizabeth. They have three grown children, Donny, Nick, and Sarah.

Order Dr. Strand's books and check out his web pages at:
www.drraystrand.com
or
www.releasingfat.com

Health Concepts
P. O. Box 9226
Rapid City, SD 57709